T0252019

Textile Progress

Abstracted and Indexed in:
Compendex
Elsevier Scopus
INSPEC
Textile Technology Index
World Textile Abstracts

Available online at:
www.tandf.co.uk/journals/
textileprogress

Published on behalf of
The Textile Institute by
Taylor and Francis

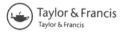
Taylor & Francis
Taylor & Francis

Typeset by Aptara, USA
Printed and bound by Hobbs the
Printers (UK), Yurchak Printing, Inc,
USA (US) or Markono (Singapore)
using the Taylor & Francis Print
On Demand model. For more
information please email
AcademicJournalsManufacturing
@informa.com

Textile Progress is a monograph series that since 1969 has provided critical and comprehensive examination of the origination and application of developments in the international fibre, textile and apparel industry and in its products.

All published research articles in this journal have undergone rigorous peer review, based on initial editor screening and anonymous refereeing by independent expert referees.

Prospective authors are invited to submit an outline of their proposed contribution for consideration by the Editor-in-Chief to: Professor Xiaoming Tao, Editor-in-Chief, Textile Progress, Institute of Textiles and Clothing, Hong Kong Polytechnic University, Hung Hom, Kowloon, Hong Kong. Email: tctaoxm@inet.polyu.edu.hk

Textile Progress

December 2011
Vol 43   No 4

Development of medical garments and apparel for the elderly and the disabled

**Ng Sau-Fun, Hui Chi-Leung
and Wong Lai-Fan**

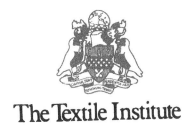

The Textile Institute

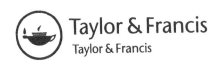

Taylor & Francis
Taylor & Francis

SUBSCRIPTION INFORMATION

Textile Progress (USPS Permit Number pending), Print ISSN 0040-5167, Online ISSN 1754-2278, Volume 43, 2011.

Textile Progress (www.tandf.co.uk/journals/TTPR) is a peer-reviewed journal published quarterly in March, June, September and December by Taylor & Francis, 4 Park Square, Milton Park, Abingdon, Oxon, OX14 4RN, UK on behalf of The Textile Institute.

Institutional Subscription Rate (print and online): $464/£244/€370
Institutional Subscription Rate (online-only): $417/£219/€333 (plus tax where applicable)
Individual members of **The Textile Institute** can subscribe to *Textile Progress* for just **£40**. Please visit http://www.tandf.co.uk/journals/offer/ttpr-so.asp for further information or contact Jacqui Tearle, Customer Services, Taylor & Francis Group, 4 Park Square, Milton Park, Abingdon, OX14 4RN, UK. Email: jacqui.tearle@tandf.co.uk.

Taylor & Francis has a flexible approach to subscriptions enabling us to match individual libraries' requirements. This journal is available via a traditional institutional subscription (either print with online access, or online-only at a discount) or as part of the Engineering, Computing and Technology Collection or S&T Library. For more information on our sales packages please visit http://www.tandfonline.com/page/librarians

All current institutional subscriptions include online access for any number of concurrent users across a local area network to the currently available backfile and articles posted online ahead of publication.

Subscriptions purchased at the personal rate are strictly for personal, non-commercial use only. The reselling of personal subscriptions is prohibited. Personal subscriptions must be purchased with a personal cheque or credit card. Proof of personal status may be requested.

Ordering Information: Please contact your local Customer Service Department to take out a subscription to the Journal: **India**: Universal Subscription Agency Pvt. Ltd, 101–102 Community Centre, Malviya Nagar Extn, Post Bag No. 8, Saket, New Delhi 110017. **USA, Canada and Mexico**: Taylor & Francis, 325 Chestnut Street, 8th Floor, Philadelphia, PA 19106, USA. Tel: +1 800 354 1420 or +1 215 625 8900; fax: +1 215 625 8914; email: customerservice@taylorandfrancis.com. **UK and all other territories**: T&F Customer Services, Informa Plc., Sheepen Place, Colchester, Essex, CO3 3LP, UK. Tel: +44 (0)20 7017 5544; fax: +44 (0)20 7017 5198; email: subscriptions@tandf.co.uk.

Dollar rates apply to all subscribers outside Europe. Euro rates apply to all subscribers in Europe, except the UK and the Republic of Ireland where the pound sterling price applies. If you are unsure which rate applies to you please contact Customer Services in the UK. All subscriptions are payable in advance and all rates include postage. Journals are sent by air to the USA, Canada, Mexico, India, Japan and Australasia. Subscriptions are entered on an annual basis, i.e. January to December. Payment may be made by sterling cheque, dollar cheque, euro cheque, international money order, National Giro or credit cards (Amex, Visa and Mastercard).

Back Issues: Taylor & Francis retains a three year back issue stock of journals. Older volumes are held by our official stockists to whom all orders and enquiries should be addressed:
Periodicals Service Company, 11 Main Street, Germantown, NY 12526, USA. Tel: +1 518 537 4700; fax: +1 518 537 5899; email: psc@periodicals.com.

The 2011 US Institutional subscription price is $450. Periodical postage paid at Jamaica, NY and additional mailing offices. **US Postmaster:** Please send address changes to TTPR, Taylor & Francis, 325 Chestnut Street, Suite 800, Philadelphia, PA 19106.

Subscription records are maintained at Taylor & Francis Group, 4 Park Square, Milton Park, Abingdon, OX14 4RN, United Kingdom.

For more information on Taylor & Francis' journal publishing programme, please visit our website: www.tandf.co.uk/journals.

CONTENTS

Textile Progress
Vol. 43, No. 4, December 2011, 235–285

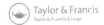

Development of medical garments and apparel for the elderly and the disabled

Ng Sau-Fun*, Hui Chi-Leung and Wong Lai-Fan

Institute of Textiles and Clothing, The Hong Kong Polytechnic University, Hung Hom, Kowloon, Hong Kong

(Received 28 February 2011; final version received 15 March 2011)

The paper critically reviews medical garments with various functions and development aspects. Textiles used and developing technologies are systematically introduced. Medical garment products are described according to three major functions: protective, treatment and caring functions. Although the main theme of this paper discusses products for the elderly and the disabled, it also contains major parts on medical garments, which include personal protective equipment (PPE), hip protectors (HP), pressure garments (PG), compression stockings (CS), wet dressings, products for wound dressing, adult incontinence products, sanitary napkins, disposable diapers, vital signs monitoring garments, motion aware clothing, wearable sensors and smart diapers and so on. The development of apparel for the elderly and the disabled is a challenge for the healthcare and clothing industries. The developed apparel products are not only based on various design, fashion and comfort concepts but also considered in terms of particular medical problems, restorative care functions and appropriate solutions for healthcare purposes.

Keywords: medical garment; adaptive clothing; dressing for the elderly and the disabled

1. Introduction

Medical garments are apparel designed for people with medical problems and/or medical personnel for the functions within protection and treatment domains. Depending on the different specific functions of medical garments, the application of appropriate medical textiles with modified designs should be adopted to tailor products for particular purposes.

Medical textiles, which are essential materials for the production of medical garments, have been developed in the past decades. A medical textile is a type of advanced technical textile and is classified according to its technical performance and functional properties as being suitable for medical or hygienic products. Many newly invented medical textiles, which have their own specific functions, have been utilized for the production of medical garments in order to achieve a higher level of medical treatment and better quality of life.

A number of reviews on medical textiles have been published, which have covered the topics of usage and details of all kinds of medical textiles and products according to their applications. A series of publications can be referred [1–5]. In this paper, literature on medical garments is systematically reviewed in the following chapter. In order to illustrate a clear picture of medical garments, an insight into their classification and development should be probed as follows.

*Corresponding author. Email: tcngsf@inet.polyu.edu.hk

ISSN 0040-5167 print/ISSN 1754-2278 online
© 2011 The Textile Institute
http://dx.doi.org/10.1080/00405167.2011.573240
http://www.tandfonline.com

1.1. Classification of medical garments

Medical garments can be classified on the basis of their specified functions. Basically, there are three main functional domains: protective, treatment and caring. The specified functions of medical garments determine the rigid requirements for designing the clothing with particular choice of appropriate medical textiles in their production. As medical garments are healthcare products with functional-oriented design, most traditional medical clothing is mainly focused on their functional values, that is, the effectiveness of the clothing to provide the required protection or clinical treatment for a certain category of patients or medical personnel. Many people find that traditional medical garments are generally embarrassing to wear. Poor fitting, comfort and appearance of a garment would make people less likely to wear it.

Corresponding to rapid exploitation in biomedical science, there is a large space for new development and modification in the design of medical garments. With a great concern, user-oriented apparel for healthcare should be produced to fulfill the requirements for restorative care training and convenient long-term nursing, as well as to provide a better ameliorant and make people more likely to want to wear them than they to the conventional medical garments.

1.1.1. Protective function domain

One of the basic functions of medical garments is to provide protection for medical personnel or patients from bacteria, physiological liquids, biological pollution and various harmful substances. Many medical garments are commercially available, of which scrubs, masks, patient gowns, surgeons' clothes and laboratory coats have played a significant role for the protection of medical teams from infection or hazardous environments. Medical garments can also have a significant impact on healing or for treatment purposes in the field of medical sciences.

1.1.2. Treatment function domain

Apart from the safety issue from infection or hazardous environments, medical garments can also have a significant impact on healing or for treatment purposes. Post-operative compression garments play a vital role in the recovery process in cosmetic surgery. For example, pressure garments (PGs) are the major treatment modalities for hypertrophic scars, and compressive stockings are commonly used for the prevention and treatment of varicose veins.

1.1.3. Caring function domain

Some users may have different types of physical impairments. Some of them may have scoliosis or kyphosis, so their body dimensions may differ from those of the stipulated pattern of medical garments in the usual production line. This group of people has reported that they have had difficulty in finding well fitting and available clothing in the current clothing market [6]. As with readymade clothes, where items which have been designed on the patterns based on size systems of norm [7] took over the current clothing market, they would also like to have access to some types of apparels for care function that fit their requirements.

Moreover, some users with physical and mental disabilities would suffer from an inability to dress themselves and would have difficulties in dressing due to their impairments.

Some of them even need long-term care and assistance in their daily life. These people or patients require some types of adapted tailored apparel to suit their special physical and psychological requirements.

Most medical garments are manufactured for protection and treatment. The symbolic value of conventional medical clothing is usually not a concern. Although functional value is of critical importance, the symbolic value of designing a garment should also be considered for meeting users' psychological needs. The symbolic values include the image, dignity and social acceptance of the user. Nobody would like to look drastically different as compared with social norms. Thus, in addition to the current needs of medical garments, some kinds of medical apparel should be designed to offer users a more dignified appearance, more encouragement for social connection and to be more appealing to wear.

As a result, some types of user-oriented apparels should be designed and produced in combination with both functional and symbolic values for treating users' current needs. The important criteria [6] for functional and symbolic values regarding clothing design are as follows:

- *Functional values*: Protection, care, comfort and ease of dressing.
- *Symbolic values*: Self-esteem, group membership, decoration and fashion.

These deliverables would help users with medical problems in enhancing their independent living, self-worth and social acceptance.

1.2. Development of medical garments

In the past decades, the demand for medical products has gradually increased due to the rapid growth in the elderly population. As a result of obtaining more knowledge in health and receiving better medical services, people's lifespan has increased. Healthcare expenditure on medical garments in the global market is going to increase continuously. This would give an impetus to the development of new medical garments. An overview of the historical development of medical garments can give us a clear tendency that leads to its future prospect.

1.2.1. Historical development of medical garments

The traditional applications of medical textiles, such as wipes and swabs, gauzes, bandages, wound dressings, surgical wear, masks, orthopedic applications and light support and compression garments, have been diversely utilized by mass population and healthcare professionals. Depending upon different applications of these medical and healthcare products, medical garments can be broadly divided into the following categories [2]: (1) healthcare hygiene products; (2) extracorporeal devices; (3) therapeutic products; (4) implantable materials; and (5) non-implantable materials.

- *Healthcare hygiene products*: These are the primary healthcare products for protection and general hygiene, and include bedding clothing, mattress covers, surgical gowns, face masks, head and shoe covers, apparel, sterilization wraps, incontinence care pads, nappies, tampons and so forth.
- *Extracorporeal devices*: These are used for supporting functions of vital organs such as kidney, liver, lung, heart pacer and so forth.
- *Therapeutic products*: These are used for the treatment and cure of diseases due to ill health, and include heating pads.

- *Non-implantable materials*: These are used as wipes, swabs, wound dressings, bandages, gauzes, plasters, press garments, orthopedic belts and so on.
- *Implantable materials*: These are used as implants in the human body to either support or replace the functions of internal tissues, and include sutures, heart valves, vascular grafts, artificial veins, artificial tendons and ligaments, artificial joints and bones, artificial skin, artificial cartilage and so on.

Medical garment products are diversely distributed in the categorization of non-implantable materials, hygiene products and therapeutic products, including surgical gowns, face masks, head and shoe covers, apparel, plasters and press garments. In 2002, healthcare hygiene products accounted for 78% of the mass consumption of medical garment products' sales, whereas it accounted for 14% and 8% of those products' sales in medical and industrial applications, respectively [2]. This shows that the healthcare hygiene products, which occupy a huge section of massive consuming medical garments, provide hygiene care/treatment for patients and protection for clinical professionals.

1.2.2. Trends of medical garments

Due to rapid growth in the development of manufacturing methods for technical textiles, there are numerous newly invented medical textiles for the production of medical garments. The market sales of these medical garment products are growing constantly owing to the increase in global population, improved healthcare standards and longer life spans. The demand rate of healthcare hygiene products, including diapers, adult incontinence products, feminine hygiene products, fabric softener and care wipers, is increasing rapidly in the market because these are widely used in the medical, hygiene and healthcare sectors.

1.2.3. Future scope of medical garments

The market demands for medical garment products will not only increase but will also become more sophisticated and environment-friendly. The conventional medical garments have numerous improved spaces in the aspects of wearer comfort, convenience in dressing, discreet designs in pattern outlook and in-built sensors for health monitoring.

Newly invented medical textiles have propelled recent advances and future trends in medical garments. More and more innovations in medical garments are developed with the incorporation of microprocessors or piezo-electrodes as part of their functionality or performance.

With the rapid growth in global population, demands for providing better healthcare to cope with modern health hazards have become more and more popular; therefore, the future development will trace and explore innovation of wearer comfort functional garments.

2. Review of medical garments for protective function

Extensive literature reviews are presented in this chapter and the following chapters on the function-related topics of medical garments under three domains: (1) personal protective equipment (PPE) and hip protector (HP) for protective function; (2) PGs and compression stockings (CS) for treatment function; and (3) care apparel and hygiene products for care function. The review is a comprehensive piece of all studies and interpretation of literature, and relates to the respective domains of medical garments from relevant journal papers, books and Internet publications. A number of issues regarding the specific functions of medical garments, which lead to the development of new insights in each domain, have been identified and discussed.

Theoretically, protection is one of the main functions of clothing. All clothing is protective to some extent. The degree of protection from a specific hazard is the major concern for selecting suitable protective clothing. Wearing suitable clothes makes wearers comfortable. They also provide protection from danger or injury, and keep them healthy and safe. Protective clothing refers to garments and other fabric-related items designed to protect the wearer from harsh environmental effects that may result in injuries or death [8]. Protective clothing is manufactured using traditional textile manufacturing technologies such as weaving and knitting and also by specialized techniques such as 3D weaving and braiding by using natural and man-made fibers [9].

Protective textiles are a part of technical textiles and comprise all those textile-based products that are used principally for their performance or functional characteristics rather than their aesthetic or decorative characteristics [10]. Textiles are an integral part of most protective equipment. Depending on the end-use, personal protective textiles can be classified as industrial protective textiles, agricultural protective textiles, military protective textiles, civilian protective textiles, medical protective textiles, sports protective textiles and space protective textiles [11]. A wide variety of PPE is manufactured to suit particular end-use requirement with relevant personal protective textiles. Medical garments with protective functions, such as PPE to protect healthcare workers (HCWs) and frail patients in potentially hazardous healthcare settings, or HP to provide injury prevention and protection for pelvic health, are produced with innovative materials and technologies and are capable of meeting user needs.

2.1. Medical drapes and gowns

All medical workers and HCWs are in touch with patients during medical procedures. They are likely to be exposed to different infections and microorganisms, which can cause disease transmission if sufficient protection is not provided in healthcare settings or in the work environment. Medical drapes and gowns are typical medical protective clothing that play an important role in minimizing disease transmission and protecting both medical professionals from coming into contact with infectious materials or pathogens and patients from possible contamination. These are outer garments to be worn in occupational exposure conditions in which blood or other potentially infectious materials may pass through and reach the HCWs' clothes and skin [12].

Medical drapes and gowns could be classified as disposable, limited use and reusable garments on the basis of their service life [13]. A disposable medical garment cannot be cleaned or reused after a single use. Some medical drapes and gowns can be cleaned and maintained for reserving only for a limited usage. It becomes unusable when it is heavily soiled or damaged after being used for several times. Reusable medical garments are designed for repeated cleaning and for providing reasonable durability with acceptable performance. All types of medical drapes and gowns would be rendered unusable if they are damaged on being used or contaminated during medical procedures.

2.1.1. Textile materials for medical drapes and gowns

The basic requirements of textile materials for producing medical drapes or gowns are their liquid barrier performance and breathability. There are other factors, such as tearing strength, abrasion resistance and sterile concerns, that would influence the selection of appropriate textile materials for medical drapes and gowns. The ideal material should be an efficient liquid barrier with high breathable properties, which could prevent the transmission of microorganisms from nonsterile to sterile areas.

A major source of contamination in wards or surgical rooms is lint from fabrics used in clothing or wipers [14–18]. Lints are very short and fine fibers that come off the fabric surface. As lint from clothing may act as a carrier of microbes, bacteria and viruses and may infect wounds, this could increase the risk of nosocomial infection and foreign body reactions. These unwanted particles from medical drapes and gowns might complicate the wound healing process [19]. Therefore, sterile lint-free drapes and gowns should be worn in surgical rooms that can help to preserve sterile or aseptic conditions, protect medical personnel from pathogens originating from patients and also protect patients from bacterial transmissions from medical personnel [20].

In the late 1990s, Goad and Taylor [21] developed a tightly woven fabric for medical clothing in a plain weave pattern. This lint-free medical fabric is made from 100% polyester yarns and treated with flame-resistant, water repellent and antimicrobial finish. New surgical textiles with improved qualities have been continuously developed after the 1990s. For example, DuPont has developed a series of protective garments using gown fabric of trademark Tyvek IsoClean [22], which could provide an inherent barrier to particles, microorganisms and nonhazardous light liquid splash. Their fabric is made of polyethylene (PE) and coated with spun-bonded polypropylene (PP) using a patented flash spinning process. Woven or nonwoven PE is commonly used for making surgical drapes and gowns to minimize cross-infection and provide a very high level of protection for HCWs [23]. Softesse medical fabric is a comfortably soft fabric for gowns and drapes and can provide acceptable barrier protection against liquid penetration [24].

Medical drapes and gowns made from PP material with a coating of PE are also commonly used in the healthcare field. The PP material is good for making disposable medical protective garments because it is comfortable and light in weight. It is also easy for injection molding and good in dimensional stability during autoclave sterilization [25]. The PE coating provides a strong barrier to fluids and a high level of protection for HCWs.

A wide array of impervious materials is available for making single-use or reusable medical drapes and gowns. The reusable textile materials are woven fabrics, including tightly woven cotton, cotton poplin reinforced with polyester, double-layer linen cotton and fabrics made from multifilament polyester yarns. Due to the high costs of laundering and sterilization for reuse, most medical drapes and gowns nowadays are disposed of after single use, and nonwoven materials are commonly adopted for producing disposable medical garments [26]. Nonwovens made from PP fibers are commonly used for producing disposable healthcare products such as hospital gowns, uniforms and surgical gowns [27].

The three most commonly used nonwoven fabrics for surgical gowns and drapes are in structure of: (1) spunlace; (2) spunbond–meltblown–spunbond (SMS); and (3) wet-laid nonwoven fabric [28]. Spunlacing is a process that employs rows of fine high-pressure water jets for mechanical bonding, which entangles a web of loose fibers on a porous belt or a perforated screen to form a sheet structure of nonwoven fabric [29]. The spunlace technology for high-energy hydroentangling and patterning processes was developed and patents were obtained by DuPont from 1963 to 1970 [30]. Most spunlaced products are made from hydroentangled fabrics, which are consolidated by the action of water jets, forming ridges on the fabric surface [31]. Other specific terms, such as jet-entangled, water-entangled and hydroentangled or hydraulically needled, are also applied for spunlaced nonwoven materials [32]. Spunlaced materials are composed of cellulose, that is, wood pulp, or blended with polyester fibers for providing a fluid barrier and better strength.

Spunlaced materials possess unique properties of high drape, softness and comfortable handling. Therefore, these are appropriate for the production of medical gowns, medical dressings and other disposable products such as wipes [33].

Spunbond–meltblown–spunbond fabrics are produced through an extrusion process and are typically composed of PP fibers, with a layer of meltblown fiber sandwiched between the two spunbond fabric layers. The middle layer of an SMS–PP nonwoven material acts as a fluid barrier membrane to prevent the passage of bloodborne pathogens or disease-causing microbes, while two layers of spunbond fabrics are mainly used to provide fabric strength [31]. In general, meltblown nonwoven fabrics are lighter and have lower strength than spunbonded fabrics. Different techniques based on the required thickness are applied to produce meltblown webs. A thin meltblown web is bonded by means of heated calender rollers, whereas a thicker meltblown web is needled mechanically [34].

Most protective medical garments, which are used widely in medical fields, are made of three-layered SMS fabrics. Many hospital garments are made of SMS–PP nonwoven composites, in which the added barrier membranes are incorporated in the middle layer to prevent the passage of bloodborne pathogens or disease-causing microbes [35]. Additional spunbond and meltblown web layers are also used for making nonwoven composite multi-layer fabrics, for example, four layers with two layers of meltblown webs sandwiched between two layers of spunbond fabric layers, or five layers with three layers of meltblown webs sandwiched between two layers of spunbond fabric layers, or one layer of meltblown web sandwiched between four layers of spunbond fabric layers, or six layers generally composed of spunbond fabric, or seven layers composed of spunbond fabric [36]. Various compositions of spunbond and meltblown materials enable the excellent combination for the filtration and absorption property of medical protective products and can provide a more breathable and comfortable barrier for the wearer [37].

Wet-laid nonwovens are made by a modified papermaking process to produce nonwoven structures with textile–fabric characteristics. By using the wet-laid technology, the fibers to be used undergo swelling and dispersion in water [38]. Even though any natural or synthetic fiber could be used in the production of wet-laid nonwovens, synthetic fiber paper is commonly adopted for disposable medical/surgical drapes or gowns. Specialty synthetic fibers may be used to provide specialized properties. For example, synthetic wood pulp made from polyolefin fibers is used for improving wet strength; crimped synthetic fibers can provide soft and bulky properties to the nonwoven products. The properties of bonding agents used in nonwoven materials are as important as the fiber material and the web structure. It affects the strength, handle, drape and softness of the nonwoven materials. The most common bonding material used in bonding wet-laid nonwovens is a water-based emulsion or dispersion ("latex") of a cross-linkable synthetic polymer, such as a polyacrylate, styrene-butadiene polymer, ethylene-vinyl acetates, vinyl chlorides and so on. The wet-laid nonwovens are significant in filtration textiles and used widely for making disposable medical garments and other hygiene products [39,40].

Chemical finishes can be applied on nonwoven materials by the process of chemical bonding with chemical agents, such as activated carbon for odor control, antimicrobials for barrier properties and so on [41]. For example, the DuPont Sontara is a nonwoven fabric with plasma and antimicrobial finishes. In the study done by Virk et al. [42], the test result showed that this fabric had higher blood and water resistance and provided a better barrier against microbes when compared with other surgical gown fabrics with fluorocarbon finish.

For both woven and nonwoven fabrics for surgical gowns and drapes, additional materials can be added by coating, providing extra layers, reinforcement or lamination of additional materials to enhance and improve their properties and performance [43]. A study done by Hubbard et al. [44] on reducing blood contamination and injury in the operation theater has suggested that there are three types of qualified medical gowns and drapes, which are made from the following materials: (1) the "standard fabric," which is a single-layer fabric material, (2) the "reinforced fabric," with an additional second layer of fabric for reinforcement and (3) the "impervious fabric," which is reinforced with PE for provision of fluid resistance; also the "zone-impervious fabric" can provide partially liquid-proof protection.

2.1.2 Design considerations for medical gowns

Gowns should be designed to provide a continuous barrier to the anterior areas of users and should have long sleeves with tight fitting cuffs that provide an adequate overlap with gloves at the wrist and should not have seams or closures that could allow liquid penetration, particularly of blood or body fluids [45]. Medical gowns can be used as examination or isolation gowns and must be designed with long sleeves for complete protection; sleeveless gown designs are not suitable for use as isolation gowns. The current gown design is generally composed of a body portion and two separate sleeve portions. A method was invented by Scrivens [46] for bonding or affixing the sleeve portion to the main body portion of the gown with adhesives, heat, radio frequency or sonic energy according to the gowns' fabric. The current disposable medical gowns with reinforced sleeves of impervious material can reduce the risk of exposure to contamination; however, their axial seams have provided a route for potential microbial transmission. A medical gown with a tubular, seamless and impervious protective layer surrounding sleeves was designed by Lopez [47] to provide enhanced protection from contamination. The seamless impervious protective layer, which can be made from PE, is adhered to the sleeves with common adhesives.

A full set of disposable protective hospital gowns, including body portion, sleeves connected with gloves, hood portions with large front viewing opening and a protective flap covering the ventilating mask, was made by Wheeler and Germy [48] to provide a unitary structure impervious to body fluids and germs for preventing the transmission of any disease. Sealed seam design was applied between the hood and body portions, and the lower front edge of the head covering was connected with the protective gown for ease of fit, maximum comfort and protection. The back of the body of this unitary gown had a plurality of adhesive strips or Velcro fasteners in a vertical opening design and could improve the fit, provide adjustment and tighten the elastic neck portion of the gown in order to completely envelop the wearer and guarantee maximum protection from contamination.

An improved disposable surgical gown comprising a body shielding panel and sleeves was invented by Holt [49] to provide overall protection and retain air permeability for maintaining a sufficient comfort to the wearer. A fluid impermeable protection region at the front of the unitary body shielding panel was fabricated from bonded layers trilaminate, including a blood/fluid absorbent outer layer, a fluid impermeable barrier layer and a perspiration absorbent inner layer. The body shielding panel was made from a nonwoven material, which is air permeable and fluid absorbent, along with the fluid impermeable barrier fabricated from a PP material to prevent fluid permeation between inner and outer layers. The sleeves, which were constructed from bonded bilaminate materials with a fluid impermeable PP barrier layer and a fluid absorbent nonwoven inner layer, were attached to the body shielding panel for securing the gown for the wearer.

Another type of improved medical gown having adhesive closures with liquid impervious coatings at frontal chest area and sleeves regions was also developed by Taylor et al. [50] to be easy to put on and take off, and protect the wearer from contamination. The preferred coating material, that is, polyvinylchloride plastisol, or other suitable coating materials, including polyurethanes, polyetherurethanes, PEs and PPs, were used for liquid impervious coatings; these were coated on the fluid's impervious fabric. The adhesive closures comprising a piece of double-sided tape on the second side of the gown could be affixed to the first side of the gown to make it easy to put on and take off.

Nowadays, different gowns are designed for handling different surgical procedures. Commonly, four strategies, including structural analysis, sizing analysis, fabric utilization assessment and fit evaluation, are employed in design analysis for all kinds of garments [51]. A study was undertaken by Pissiotis et al. [52] to compare the barrier function, comfort and protection afforded by nine types of surgical gowns and to identify factors that may influence their effectiveness. The results of this study showed that half of all studied gowns, which were used during 250 major operations by the surgeons and assistants, became contaminated from outside. The rate of blood strikethrough was up to 90% in reusable gowns, but was only 11% in disposable single-layer gowns, and was even as low as only 3% in disposable reinforced gowns. The most vulnerable strikethrough areas were cuffs, forearms, thighs, chest and abdomen. Reinforced disposable gowns provided better protection. Most surgeons felt comfortable and protected while wearing disposable gowns, but only up to 4% of surgeons felt comfortable and safe while wearing reusable gowns.

Comfort issues of wearing are dependent on complex interactions between the permeability and flexibility of fabric, climatic, physiological and psychological variables, also related to product design [53,54]. A combination of factors, such as temperature, humidity, air movement and so forth, may influence the wearing comfort. Due to the desirable protective capability of medical gowns, air permeability would become the main determinant for wearing comfort [55]. In general, high liquid barrier performance materials for medical gowns have low air permeability, that is, the single-layer polyolefin film gowns offer maximum protection but are uncomfortable because the air permeability of such fabric is low.

There is a wide array of impervious materials used for producing gowns for their liquid barrier performance and breathability. The ideal material for gowns would be an efficient liquid barrier with a high breathable property. Single-use gowns are most commonly made from nonwoven materials alone or in combination with materials such as plastic films that offer increased protection from liquid penetration. For reusable gowns, the ability to maintain complete barrier effectiveness despite multiple washings is necessary, because these may lose barrier properties from abrasion and get damaged during wear and the breakdown of fabric during laundering and sterilization [56]. Both single-use and reusable products are commonly reinforced to enhance or improve their properties and performance. The optimal protection gown would cover the entire front of the torso and arms with plastic supplementary apron and plastic sleeves [57–59].

2.2. Hip protectors (HP)

The aging process causes degeneration of nerves, joints and muscles, and the incidence of falls becomes high in elderly people [60]. In particular, the elderly who often take numerous medications for multiple chronic diseases are found at an increased risk of falls [61]. Most hip fractures occur as a result of sideways falls, directly impacting the hip bones of proximal femurs [62,63]. Hip fractures can be devastating injuries that result in disability, functional impairment and mortality in elderly people [64–67].

Hip protectors are medical devices commonly used to reduce the risk of hip fractures from falls in elderly people who have compromised weaker bone micro-architecture and are at a high risk of falling [68,69]. Numerous scientific studies and clinical tests on HPs have shown that people are less likely to suffer from a hip fracture when wearing HPs, which can be effective in preventing hip fractures and decreasing the risk of hip injuries among the elderly [70–72].

There is a variety of HP models with different designs and made of different materials. Generally, HPs are specially designed underpants with protective shields, which were either hard shields or soft pads to be placed bilaterally along the hip to cover the greater trochanter [73,74]. On the basis of the way of installation of protective shields, HPs can be classified into two main categories: (1) underpants with sewn-in shields, and (2) underpants with detachable shields, which are inserted inside the pockets located bilaterally over vulnerable hip areas [75,76].

The sewn-in shields can be contained in close-fitting HPs and ensure that the functional part is held in the correct position to provide thorough protection to fragile hips, but not easy to notice if the shell is broken; therefore, more care and time are required during laundering and drying for this type of HP to ensure its efficiency. The HP with detachable shields is easy to wear. The protective shields can be inserted inside the bilateral pockets after putting on, and can be removed for laundering. However, the detachable shields have to be placed into the correct position to provide thorough protection to hip bones.

The functional part of HP is the protective shield, which has to be centered over the greater trochanter region and securely positioned in bilateral pockets, and has a certain degree of resilience to hold the hip pads in the relative right position with respect to vulnerable hip areas while being worn [77]. The function of these shields would effectively attenuate and shunt away the impact force created in sideways falls of the elderly from the greater trochanter region to prevent hip fractures and hip injuries through one or a combination of two mechanisms: energy-absorbing and energy-shunting systems [78,79].

There are two main types of HP products currently available in the market, namely energy-absorbing soft pads and energy-shunting hard shells, as well as the combination of these two systems, used to protect the hip area and prevent hip fractures. The principle of an energy-shunting HP is to distribute impact loads away from the greater trochanter (GT) to the surrounding soft tissues, while an energy-absorbing device attenuates impact forces by means of a shock-absorbing material [80]. Both hard shell HPs, which primarily shunt away energy, and soft-pad HPs, which primarily absorb energy, are capable of reducing the risk of a hip fracture in the falls of elderly people by nearly 60% when worn correctly, and both can be recommended to the elderly as a means of preventing hip fractures [81,82]. However, the hard shell HPs are more likely to crack or break following a fall.

Hip protectors using the combination of both principles are composed of a rigid shell made of acrylonitrile–butadiene–styrene (ABS) with a soft lining of closed-cell polyurethane. This combination pad consists of a rigid shell placed on top of a soft flexible material that is used to absorb the impact energy; the harder and stiffer shell is used to shunt the impact energy resulting from a sideways fall away from the hip bones onto the surrounding soft tissue linings [83]. The function of these combination pads can prevent the GT from coming into contact with the impact surface, and the energy absorption component will absorb a certain amount of impact energy, with the rest shunted to the pad periphery for absorption by local soft tissues. An anatomically designed energy-shunting and energy-absorbing HP can provide an effective impact force attenuation in typical falling conditions of the elderly [84]. Daners et al. [85] in an investigative study showed that the HP in an arrangement of a hard shell with soft lining had the best performance and higher force reduction than those with a foam pad or a hard shell alone [85]. No matter which type has been used, a HP should be worn at all times when the person is at risk of falling [86], as most hip fractures occur when the HPs are not used, and the effectiveness of HPs would be limited by poor compliance [87,88].

2.2.1. Textiles used for HP

Due to the accumulated intrinsic effects of aging, the skin of a frail old person can easily be at the risk of tissue breakdown and localized damage to the skin, and the underlying tissues cause the development of bedsores or pressure ulcers. The underpant textiles and padding materials, which are used for making HPs, have a considerable influence on factors, such as pressure, friction and skin hydration, which contribute to skin ulceration [89]. A durable synthetic stretch textile, such as knitted cotton–polyester blend with spandex knitted fabrics, which is commonly used for underwear, is generally adopted for making HPs in order to obtain a close fit and ensure that the protective shields are located at right positions over the vulnerable hip areas in order to achieve the optimal protection. The knitted fabrics comprise blends of cotton and synthetic fibers that possess recoverable stretch characteristics, and the production of cotton-polyester blend fabrics is knitted from standard or normal twist yarns, which have desirable stretch properties in the filling direction, and are especially appropriate for making HP [90]. Heavyweight cotton blends with polyester or spandex for manufacturing garments could maintain their elastic properties after a 52-week laundry test. This result indicated that HP, which is made from synthetic material blended with cotton and spandex, could provide reasonable durability and comfort [91]. As the textile material used for making the underpants for HP would be in contact with the wearers' skin for a long period, it is required for providing superior comfort to the wearer.

The padding materials such as HP protective shields, which are sewn-in or detachable, are inserted strategically inside pockets sandwiching in-between the underpants garment, and are currently either a soft pad of curved, dense foam or a rigid PP grill in round or oval shapes. The first HP padding material, which was made of a special silicone rubber, was proposed by Wortberg [92] as early as in 1988. Since then, another material, such as PE foam [93], is used as the padding material; some models consisted of an outer shield of PP and inner part of plastazote [94], which is a soft and resilient material with a closed cellular structure and low weight. Practically, the selected padding materials for HPs should have a good energy absorbing capacity, be high impact and shock-proof, have good durability, light weight, good recovery after compression, easy availability and reasonable cost [95]. A study was undertaken by Honkanen et al. [91] to determine why HPs with soft pads in garments of light neutral colors and cotton blend fabrics were most preferred.

2.2.2. Design considerations for improvement on the compliance

Even though wearing an HP is an effective measure for the prevention of hip fractures in the elderly, poor compliance or adherence while using HP has been recognized as a major concern in interpreting findings on HP efficacy in most of the studies [96–98]. Many previous studies showed that long-term adherence for wearing HPs was very low at about 35% [99,100]. The compliance may vary between different types of HPs.

The most frequently given reasons for nonacceptance or nonadherence of HP were general discomfort, poor fitting, poor appearance, extra effort and time to wear, and toilet difficulties [101–103]. Several studies have identified adverse effects associated with HP use and caused skin irritation [104]. Some reports indicated that the difficulties encountered by seniors in toilets were related to their physical restrictions such as muscle weakness or dementia [105,106]. The seniors with dementia had often removed the protective shield as a result of their poor cognitive function [107]. In a comparison of adherence between soft pads and hard-shelled HPs, a study was undertaken by Bentzen et al. [108] to show that the probability of a continued use of soft pad HPs was a little higher than the use of hard shelled HPs. Other studies had reported that hard-shelled HPs were too prominent and uncomfortable to wear, and also too hard to lie down on while sleeping. On the contrary, HPs with soft foam pads may be more comfortable to the subjects' skin for wearing and more acceptable for users to lie down than the rigid shield designs [109].

Some improvements, such as better fitting and appearance of the garment, should be attempted to improve comfort and increase the percentage of acceptable fit for the users [110]. The size of HP is another crucial concern for their design improvement. Some elderly expressed dissatisfaction with the limited sizes of available HPs [111]. As the body shapes of elderly people would have great variance, the conventional standardized size specification may not be appropriate, and the commercial size range is quite limited. Oversized HPs may fail to anchor the protective shield in a proper position when the wearer falls down, while an undersized HP would be too tight and cause discomfort to the user. Tailor-made HPs based on individual size and body shape could be considered for solving the fitting problems, and the appearance of an HP can be more acceptable if it looks similar to conventional male and female underpants [73]. Woo et al. [96] had suggested in his study that the body build of elderly Chinese and the hot and humid climate in Hong Kong should be considered for the design improvement of HPs [96]. Tight-fit clothing pressure should also be accurately measured for the production of HPs to obtain the best fit of the fabric to the body for the safest protection and providing a more comfortable feeling to the elderly wearing HPs [112].

Other problems of using HPs were indicated in the study done by van Schoor et al. [113], which showed that not everyone was correctly wearing the device. Some participants were wearing the device backwards or even wearing a device that had been damaged by wrong laundering, and most participants were not wearing the HP during the night [113]. Therefore, the protective shields with an appropriate thickness of effective material should be held in a correct position by being contained in a close-fitting pocket on a garment without bulgy appearance, and the shields' design should also be adjusted, making them more comfortable to wear during sleep in order to increase compliance rates [114]. In addition, the front and the back side of the HP, and the correct positions of detachable shields should be clearly marked in order to be placed properly, so that it can be worn correctly with optimal protection [115].

The HP design could be adapted for various needs of the users. A HP model with pull-up handles at the waistline can enhance independence in the elderly with arthritis or weakened grip-strength so that the HP can be easily put on without assistance [116]. An HP design with a totally open crotch allows the wearer to use the toilet easily without the necessity to take the device down and pull back up [117]. HPs fastened by a snap or Velcro could enable the caregivers to take care of people with incontinence more easily [118].

An innovative concept of using an airbag system has been suggested for HP development [119]. The airbag system was embedded in a motion sensor-based belt, which was worn by the elderly. In case of a fall, the sensors in the belt would trigger the inflation of airbags in a few milliseconds like automobile airbags. New HP designs are successively being developed and the current products are being modified to better models to address users' different needs. The efficacy of these new designs and the modified models would need to be examined under strict laboratory conditions. In addition, their effectiveness should be evaluated through the clinically controlled trials and compliance should be assessed in future research.

3. Review of medical garments for treatment function

Some medical garments are designed for the clinical treatment and cure of diseases. The use of medical garments for pressure therapy is not new in the field of rehabilitation. For example, the use of PG for preventing hypertrophic scarring and the use of CSs for managing chronic venous ulcers are well known. Another application of medical garments for treatment function is wet dressing, which is used to relieve symptoms of some skin diseases.

3.1. Pressure garments (PGs)

Pressure garments, which are also known as compression garments, are tight-fitting garments made of elastic materials. Hypertrophic scars are thickened, hard areas of scar tissues, which are commonly the result of thermal, electrical and chemical burns when the skin is damaged beyond a critical depth. If the skin is severely damaged down to the recticular dermis, the papillary dermis normal pressure would be destroyed and hypertrophic scars would occur due to overgrowth of scar tissue. Hypertrophic scarring may result in cosmetic disfigurement, pruritus, skin hypersensitivity, joint contractures and functional disability [120,121]. Functional and cosmetic disability can be quite marked, depending on the site of injury and the extent of damage. Pressure therapy has proven highly successful in preventing severe hypertrophic scar formation [122]. PGs are worn to exert pressure over wounded areas to help the skin heal smoothly in order to avoid scarring that would otherwise occur [123–125].

The range of pressure found to be of therapeutic value in the management of hypertrophic scars lies between 10 mmHg (1.3 kPa) and 35 mmHg (45 kPa). In the clinical study conducted by Naismith [126], scars treated with pressure in excess of 15 mmHg appeared flatter, smoother and less erythematous than scars subjected to lower pressure. However, the applied pressure should never be beyond the upper acceptable boundary; pressure greater than 40 mmHg (5.2 kPa) will result in maceration and even paraesthesia. The optimum amount of pressure required to prevent hypertrophic scarring is still subject to disagreement. In general, PGs are designed to exert a pressure of approximately 25 mmHg on the underlying tissue [127].

PGs should be applied as soon as the wound site is healed. The period of 1–24 weeks after the injury is critical in the treatment and control of hypertrophic scarring [128]. PGs should be worn continuously, night and day, except for short periods of personal hygiene, until the scar fades or matures [129]. The length of time required for wearing the garment for treatment varies from several weeks up to about 18–24 months [130], depending on the severity of the injury and the scar maturation rate. Although ready-to-wear PGs are available, in order to provide each individual patient with correct continuous pressure over the scar area involved, PGs are generally made according to individual size and needs.

Haq and Haq [131] investigated the effectiveness of PG therapy for hypertrophic scar treatment; the result of their study showed that over 50% improvement was made to obviate the need for repetitive surgery and no recurrence was observed after the application of PG therapy. PGs are used not only for the treatment and prevention of hypertrophic scarring but also accepted to be effective and safe for the treatment of lymphedema following breast carcinoma therapy [132,133].

3.1.1. Textiles used for PG

Pressure garments currently used for the treatment of hypertrophic scars are made from different elastic fabrics with a wide range of tensions [134,135]. Normally, most PGs are made from elastic fabric containing Lycra in net structure. PGs can also be made of Tubigrip [136], which is made from cotton with covered elastic threads laid into the fabric to form free-moving spirals, and are manufactured in tubular lengths of different diameters. The different levels of elasticity and strength of the material will provide varying degrees of fabric tension, thus inducing different degrees of pressure on patients.

Patients in different phases of the healing process need PGs for different levels of pressure. Hospitals have their own operating systems. For example, three types of elastomeric Lycra fabrics with different tensile properties would be used for producing PGs in most of the hospitals in Hong Kong [137]. Children or patients with newly healed wounds or tender skin will be offered the garments made from the softest and most comfortable materials, while the stronger and greater compression materials will be used for higher compression for the late-stage healed wounds or on tough skin areas, but some hospitals use only one type of elastomeric fabric every time. Different degrees of compression produced by the PGs for different groups of patient can be achieved by adjustment of the pattern size and the PG fitting.

A number of different stretchable fabrics are used for the manufacturing of PGs. In the 1970s, Webb Associates in conjunction with the Jobst Institute [138] developed a special bobbinet and power-net fabrics for the construction of pressure gradient garments. Their fabrics were made of Spandex or rubber and Dacron/nylon blend [139]. The elastic fabric structure was designed to provide tri-dimensional control by using unidirectional tension threads wrapped with prestressed fibers and caught with bias lacing.

In England, a kind of power-net fabric, which is a warp knitted from nylon and elastane yarns, is the most popular fabric structure used in the manufacture of PGs [140]. Warp-knitted fabrics with Powernet and Sleeknit structures of polyester or polyamide and elastane are the main materials used in the manufacturing of PGs [141]. The proportions and weight of elastane in the power-net or sleeknit fabric largely determine its potential tension. PGs made of different kinds of elastomeric fabrics with different degrees of elasticity and strength of materials might provide varying compression on patients according to their requirements.

Most commercial companies would develop their own material for PGs. For example, Bioconcepts PGs are available for different parts of body with six types of materials [142]. They use regular materials for adults and children of age 11 years and older. Close-knit fabric is fine for 10-year-old children and under or for elderly patients of age 75 years and older; soft material is very light and smooth for patients with extremely sensitive skin; a soft lining is added inside the PG for sensitive areas such as elbows, axillae and knees, and insert material can be applied to irregular surfaces and concave body areas such as the axilla, hand, clavicle, neck and face [143]. A medical-grade silicone elastomer sheet, named Silon-TEX, is bonded to a Lycra spandex fabric to treat troublesome hypertrophic and keloid scars. The Medical Z's PGs [144] are made from fabrics that are compatible with oil and lotions.

Apart from the standard fabric [145] used for the treatment of edema, hypertrophic scars or keloids, CoolMax fabric [146] is used to make PGs more breathable and comfortable. PGs from Barton-Carey Medical Products [147] are made of spandex and nylon fabric. They can provide high compression of up to 50 mmHg for the treatment of lymphedema.

No matter which type of fabric is used for the making of PGs, they should be breathable, nonabrasive, durable and comfortable to wear. The tensile properties of the elastic fabric should be strong enough to provide the required compression and should enable the PG to fit the wound areas like a second skin without obstructing the body movements of patients.

3.1.2. Considerations on the design of PGs

In order to achieve the precise compression according to the clinical requirements, the PG has to be cut and sewn to an appropriate size, based on the tensile properties of the elastic fabric and the body size of individual patient. Generally, PGs are made up in three-dimensional shapes, and most of them are in tubular form. The relative size of PG to body size is reduced by a certain percentage, thus skin and garment interfacial pressure would be produced when the PG is being stressed to produce compression on the body. The "reduction percentage" of PG mainly depends on the tensile properties of the elastic fabric, the curvature of the contoured body surface and the amount of skin and the required garment interfacial pressure. On the basis of the principle of the Laplace law, Ng and Hui [148] developed a pressure model to predict the skin and garment interfacial pressure induced by different sizes of PGs on a particular curved surface of the human body. Macintyre [149] also proposed a scientific method to design PGs for human forearms and thighs. In order to increase the versatility of the design and improve the functionality of the garment, a PG may be made up of more than one layer of elastic fabric and fabrics of various tensile properties may be sewn together. Double-layered PGs are sometimes used for the application of higher pressure [150]. The skin and garment interfacial pressure for a multilayer fabric tube with the varying tensile properties of its elastic fabric could also be estimated by a theoretical model [151]. All the existing models are based on a static condition. The change in skin and garment interface pressure under body movement and mobility is not considered. Further development on the prediction of skin and garment interfacial pressure becomes necessary in dynamic situations. In addition, the effects of the percentage of body fat, skin stiffness, age and so forth on the skin and garment interface pressure are not clearly known. Different body characteristics may affect the precision of the interface pressure produced by the PG; thus, further research on these aspects would improve the accuracy of the prediction of skin and garment interface pressure.

Elastic fabrics used to make PGs are normally cut in various sizes and different aspect ratios (i.e., width of the fabric divided by the gauge length). The resultant pressure of a tubular PG exerted on a contoured body surface may vary if the load–strain relationship measured from the elastic fabric might vary with the aspect ratio [152]. In the making of PGs, different aspect ratios of elastic fabrics with biaxial extension properties should be taken into account, but the change of aspect ratios for an elastic fabric below 2.5 will not significantly affect the skin and garment interfacial pressure on human body [153]. As the compression provided by PG at the hem edges deteriorates, in order to apply the precise skin and garment interfacial pressure to the patient, the size of PG should extend at least 5 cm beyond the margins of the scar(s) [154,155].

The fabrics containing elastane yarn would suffer from the disadvantage of having a viscoelastic response to an applied load. If such fabrics are under tension over a period, some of their stress will be relieved with a consequent reduction in the skin and garment interfacial pressure. In general, slackening would occur in PGs when worn for a long time because the tension of the fabrics is time-dependent. Work done by Cheng et al. [156] demonstrated that there is a gradual decline in skin and garment interfacial pressure when patients wear PGs over a period. The elastic deterioration happening in the stretch fabric would definitely affect the clinical effectiveness of PGs. The rate of tension decay of each elastic fabric mainly depends on its properties as well as the amount and direction of stretch applied on the fabric [157]. The PGs fittings must be checked regularly by rehabilitation therapists, at least every three months, to ensure appropriate compression and comfort provided by the prescribed PGs, because these devices can normally last for 2–3 months before being stretched out [158]. The stress relaxation and shrinkage properties of different fabrics used commonly to make PGs were examined in the work of Ng-Yip [159]. The result of this study showed that shrinkage of elastic fabrics varied significantly and this should be considered in the making of PGs, but fabric shrinkage also appears to be beneficial as it compensates for loss in elasticity during washing and hence helps in maintaining a more constant fabric compression throughout the life of the PG.

The seam and stitches used in PG would affect the garment appearance, comfort and durability. Not only the appropriate type of seam and stitches must be chosen but also other sewing parameters, such as stitch tension, stitch density, size and type of sewing thread used for producing PGs, are important to the seam quality. Poor appearance and construction of PGs would cause embarrassment and other problems to patients leading to low compliance with the treatment [160,161]. The human body with its varying contours would make an uneven distribution of pressure. It is difficult to apply pressure evenly on the concave areas or at the flexor joints [162–164] of the human body. Conforming inserts made of elastomer or isoprene are commonly used as adjuncts to PGs on such irregular surface areas [165,166].

There are many other problems, such as fitting, comfort, appearance, full movement, swelling of extremities, rashes and blistering, which are associated with the use of PGs [167] and would cause poor compliance with the treatment [168]. The findings in the work of Brown [169] revealed that comfort, ease of movement and appearance were the most significant factors of compliance.

Wearing comfort is basically determined by garment fit, fabric extensibility and garment design. The pressure is the most important factor affecting the wearer's sensation of wearing comfort with this tight-fitting garment. In general, the fitting of PGs mainly relies on the experience of medical personnel or therapists. The pressure delivered by PGs is not measured objectively with any instrument. If the fitting of PGs is inappropriate, some of the pressure exerted by PGs may be too low and not potentially effective, while the rest may be too high and dangerous to the patient. The work of Williams et al. [170] showed that improvements could be made through garment design and selected fabrics. Factors such as ease of cleaning, ease of putting on/taking off and life of garment also should not be neglected.

3.2. Compression stockings (CSs)

Compression stockings, also known as graduated CSs, medical gradient stockings, medical leg wear, embolism stockings, varicose stockings, compression tights or support stockings [171], are specially designed elastic tights for exerting steady pressure on the legs to help blood flow through the veins and back to the heart that can improve circulation [172]. Medical compressive stockings have been used for many years as a mechanical pressure method for deep vein thrombosis prophylaxis and treatment of varicose veins, deep vein thrombosis, recurrence of leg ulceration and control of lymphoedema.

One of the most common clinical manifestations of venous insufficiency is the varicose veins or varicosities. Varicose veins are swollen veins that range from small "spider veins" to thick, bulging and tangled veins that can protrude beyond the skin surface [173]. The "spider veins" are fine red or blue lines just underneath the skin surface, while serious varicose veins may have a bulging and twisted look with dark blue or purple color. Varicose veins is not a cosmetic concern. It can cause a wide range of symptoms, including itching, fatigue, rash, bleeding when scratching, cramps and leg swelling, or even severe pain during standing or walking. Varicose veins commonly appear on the backs of the calves or inwardly on the legs [174]. The functional abnormalities of the venous system may lead to more advanced diseases, including venous claudication, edema, skin changes and venous ulceration [175]. The nonactive and resting elderly or patients are more susceptible to these problems.

Compression textiles are used to increase blood flow in the venous system [176–178] and to improve peripheral circulation and venous return [179,180]. Medical CSs made from elastic fabric materials are widely used as a conservative nonsurgical treatment for such problems because of its inexpensiveness and ease to apply.

3.2.1. Textiles for CSs

Generally, CSs are manufactured with wrapping elastic fibers or rubber around the stockings. The fabric's elasticity will determine its ability to resist any change in its configuration and to return to its original length, shape or size immediately after the removal of stretching force. The degree of elasticity is dependent on the textiles used and the weave of the material [181]. Compressive stockings made from fabrics of different elasticities produce different skin pressure gradient distribution, which would significantly influence the patient's venous hemodynamics [182,183]. The gradient pressure function provided by the CSs is predominately related to the structural characteristics and material properties of the stocking fabric. The work of Liu et al. [184] showed that material properties in the wale direction would exert a significant impact on the skin pressure gradient performances. Moreover, the greater extensibility and smoother surface of the fabric in the wale direction would contribute to the ease of putting the stocking on. In addition, the extension–flexion movements of the wearer's leg would also be facilitated. A supplier has developed a material by combining the Z Grip fabric with CoolMax fabric [185] for producing a type of grip stockings that can resolve the "slippery" problems of compressive stockings.

A variety of different synthetic elastomers and weaving methods have been adopted in the production of CS. Most of the fabrics are weft-knitted structures. Three fundamental stitches, including plain stitch, tuck stitch and miss-stitch, are commonly used in knitted stocking fabrics. Highly sophisticated polyesters, polymers and synthetic spandex are used for the manufacturing of CSs. These newest materials also afford extra comfort for prolonged use [186]. The different proportion of materials, including polyamide, elastomeric or gommures fibers, determine the formation of different compression levels that would be provided by the CSs [184].

Special silver fibers are woven into the materials for producing silver CSs, which could convey some natural antimicrobial protection. Functionally, such medical stockings act in lowering the risk of infection, particularly in patients who have already begun to develop ulcers on their legs [187].

3.2.2. Considerations on the application of CSs

Graduated compression is produced and distributed with different levels over the entire length of CS on the underlying skin and tissues. The maximum compression is graduated at the ankle and is gradually decreased along the length to achieve relative less tight fit at knee/thigh of the leg [188]. Special attention should be paid on the ankle part, where the pressure is relatively stronger than the other regions of the leg. The compression gradient may adversely affect the results of the applied therapy if the CSs do not fit on the leg. Compressive stockings are worn to provide sustained pressure on the limbs for longer periods and can be worn throughout the day. As repeated washing and wearing would cause loss in elasticity, CSs are probably replaced after few months of therapy.

The quality of CSs is normally measured according to their tightness exerted on legs rather than their material composition. CSs are considered as medical devices and are generally available in different levels of compression. Appropriate CSs of suitable compression should be used depending on the severity of medical conditions. The degree of pressure exerted on the skin and underlying tissues can be measured and used to grade the compression class of the stockings. However, the pressure classification may be varied and has different standards. There are two main standards of compression classes for CS: the British standard and the European standard. The British standard classified compression into the following three classes: "light compression," "medium compression" and "strong compression" within the range of 14–35 mmHg gradient pressure. The levels of gradual compression recommended by the European standard are stronger than the British standard [189]. The European standard classified compression into the following four classes: "light compression," "medium compression," "strong compression" and "heavy compression." The lowest gradient pressure recommended by the European standard is 18 mmHg and the maximum compression can be up to 59 mmHg.

CSs with light compression are used for mild varicose veins, venous hypertension in pregnancy or just for helping to relieve heaviness and fatigue in legs. The most frequently used medical CSs start from "medium" class. The "strong" class will be chosen for the severe defects of veins, while the "heavy" class will be used in the cases of lymphoedema and lipodermatosclerosis [190]. CSs are normally available in various styles [191], ranging from knee-length (atopic dermatitis, AD), thigh-length (AG) or waist-length/pantyhose (AT) in open toe, closed toe or ultra sheer designs with a wide range of opacities, colors and sizes that are virtually indistinguishable from regular hosiery or standard stockings, though they may be double the thickness of regular pantyhose [192].

Although CSs are always the first-line measures to be used for the treatment of medical problems associated with varicose veins or venous reflux, they can not eliminate the underlying clinical problems. A combination of correction measures, including exercise and weight control, avoiding prolonged standing, the application of external laser treatment, injection sclerotherapy, radiofrequency obliteration and surgery, has been applied for the treatment of varicose veins during the past several decades [193–195].

3.3. Wet dressings

Wet dressings, also known as wet-wraps or wet compresses, can be applied as compresses of moist dressings on skin. Repeated compresses of moist dressings can relieve symptoms of either acute or chronic skin conditions such as crusting, oozing and swollen or pruritic dermatoses [196]. Wet dressings are very useful for diverse types of AD [197,198], which is the common form of eczema [199], when the condition has not responded to the first-line treatment consisting of emollients and topical corticosteroids [200]. They can also improve hydration for dry lichenified lesions on skin and are useful in the management of other dry skin conditions (xerosis) such as icthyosis vulgaris. They can also be an extremely effective treatment for acute itchy skin rashes [201]. In most instances, the wet dressings are two to three layers of moist clean gauze sheeting, which are wetted with the cool salt solution, Burow's solution (Domeboro astringent solution) or acetic acid (vinegar solution), and wrapped on the affected area of the patient's skin [202]. The use of single-layer tubular bandages or dampened garments to control widespread AD is also very common.

3.3.1. Functions of wet dressings

Wet dressings can be cool, warm or at normal room temperature. Cool wet compresses are useful for cooling acute inflamed skin, decreasing pruritus and suppressing swelling by slowing the flow of blood and sera to the affected area. Warm wet compresses are useful for chronic conditions. It helps soften dried blood and sera and causes relaxation of blood vessel and connective tissues that can increase blood circulation and resolve inflammation. Wet dressings at room temperature are useful for removing crusts and adherent eschars. It could help to clean the skin's surface and provide gentle debridement [203].

Proper hydration of skin can offset xerosis, minimize exacerbations of AD and help to break the "itch-scratch" cycle. Wet-wrap treatment with emollients or corticosteroid dilutions can help to reduce pruritus and inflammation by cooling of the skin, and increase penetration of topical corticosteroids so that steroid absorption can reach both the superficial and deep layers of inflamed skin [204]. As the moisture of wet dressing evaporates, the cooling sensation on the skin has an anti-inflammatory effect and suppresses itching that can provide relief from the heat and itching sensation of eczema. Dryness on skin can be prevented as the skin can be rehydrated by the large amounts of emollients under wet dressing. As wet dressing covers and protects the skin, it can prevent damages caused by fingernails and scratching [205], and provide some protection from allergens and bacteria.

3.3.2. Textiles used for wet dressings

The use of wet dressings generally encompasses wet lightweight tubular bandages, which are made from 100% pure cotton. Dampened cotton T-shirts have also been used for dressing retention since 1970 [206]. Cotton is the most commonly used material for wet dressing due to its unique properties of excellent moisture absorption and better heat conduction. Other fibers such as wool or synthetic fabrics may cause itching, skin irritation and allergy. However, the structure of cotton contains short fibers, which expand and contract and can cause a rubbing movement to irritate delicate skin. The traditionally used cotton material is also prone to bacterial and fungal attack and the interaction of some other textiles may lead to allergic contact dermatitis. Silver fabrics or enclosed silver ions are used in medical textiles to provide protection to skin against microbial corrosion, prevention of malodor, prophylaxis and therapy of AD [207–209].

The efficacy and functionality of silver-coated textiles have been examined by previous studies [210,211] and the results showed that the silver-coated textiles could be safely used to reduce the clinical severity of AD. It showed more comfort in wearing and was functionally more effective for lessening pruritus comparable to cotton. It was also found that clothes made of these silver-coated textiles have to be worn tightly on the skin to ensure interaction between fibers and the skin. It might be sufficient to sustain a constant impairment of *Staphylococcus aureus* (*S. aureus*) growth. *S. aureus* colonization of the skin induces severe AD and often becomes infected. Therefore, the antimicrobial properties of silver-coated clothes can significantly reduce the burden of *S. aureus* and lead to a positive effect on AD when wearing silver-coated clothes overnight [212].

A number of silver-coated textile products are currently available on the market. For example, Shieldex is also known as Padycare textiles, which consist of micromesh material containing woven silver filaments with a silver content of 20% [213]. Microair Dermasilk [214] is a type of sericin-free antimicrobial silk product. It is made of transpiring and slightly elastic woven silk coated with the compound alkoxysilane quaternary ammonium, which has a durable antimicrobial finish in the textile products to prevent odor, the electron-dense granules and cytoplasm survival of bacteria, including S. aureus [212]. Sericin, a macromolecular gum-like protein on raw silk filaments, is a major component of raw silk when combined with another protein named fibroin [215]. Sericin can induce proliferation of several human cells and can be removed by the treatment called degumming during raw silk production at the reeking mill to produce a type of sericin-free lustrous and semi-transparent silk [216]. Dermasilk has no sericin and has a permanently bonded microbial agent. It has beneficial effects and can alleviate symptoms of AD on the skin. It can also be used for skin care and dressing in the management of AD [217]. The combination of sericin-free silk fabrics with silver-coated antimicrobial finish may become an ideal textile for AD patients [218].

The silver ion on silver-coated textiles is biologically active. The released silver ions can rapidly interact with chloride and proteins on the skin surface or in wound exudate and lose the antibacterial activity [211]. Another type of antimicrobial textile, which is coated or impregnated with silver nanoparticles, claims to have advantages over normal textiles, as it has properties to inhibit growth of bacteria and fungi. This nanosilver-based smart textile can be used for medical clothing, including wet-wrap garments.

Nowadays, a variety of new bandages and garments with different trade names have become available in the market. Tubegauz is a two-layer, open-weaved cotton tubular dressing with one layer impregnated with hydrocortisone cream. Another dry layer applied over the top of wet layer for wet dressings was initially reported by Goodyear et al. in 1991 [219]. Lyocell, which is a cellulosic fiber superior to cotton, provides better comfort to patient [220]. Damp Lyocell pyjamas can be used for extensive skin infections during nighttime.

The open-weave tubular stretchy Tubifast bandages are the most commonly used wet dressings. Tubifast bandages with the composition of 86% viscose, 11% nylon and 3% elastane have been used for wet and dry wrapping since 1995 [221]. Tubifast garments were introduced onto the market in 2003 [222]. Tubifast garments consist of long-sleeved roll-neck T-shirts and pull-up leggings, which are specially designed with external seams to avoid irritancy and can be used in the wet wrapping process [223]. The effectiveness of Tubifast garments for wet-wrap procedure was examined in the study done by Hon et al. [224]. It is concluded that the garments were effective in the short-term improvement of severe AD and quality of life in AD patients. There are many other brands and suppliers in the market such as Actifast (Activa), Comfifast (Shiloh Healthcare), Elastus Tubiquick (Most Active Health Care), Zipsocs, Coverflex (Hartmann) and so on [206]. There may be variations in trade names and their availability in different countries.

3.3.3. Limitations of wet dressings

Although wet dressings can be beneficial for the treatment of AD, one of their disadvantages is high cost. The cost of treatment by wet dressings is expensive, especially when the wet dressing products are only suitable for single use. For the types of reusable bandages or garments for wet dressing, most of them can be washed and reused for some time. All wet wraps should be removed or changed when they are dried, or the compresses should be remoistened periodically by squirting the solution underneath the dressings with a bulb syringe. Otherwise, the dry-out dressings may become useless. It would also make the patient feel uncomfortable and cause irritation, including hot, dry and itchy sensation to the skin [225].

Previous studies [226,227] have reviewed the efficacy and safety of web-wrap dressings. There was a concern that wet wraps used with topical corticosteroids would induce a risk for increased absorption of topical corticosteroids, which may cause adverse effects on patients' health. Practitioners trained in its use should only employ wet dressings. Specialized nursing care by a trained nurse or a committed carer is essential, especially when using wet dressing treatment for long periods [228]. Another common side effect of wet wrapping is chilling in air-conditioned environments, or in cold weather during winter. Hon et al. [224] identified other issues, such as the appearance on wearing the garment and concerned compliances, in their study.

4. Review of apparel products for caring function

Some medical apparel products are applied on the elderly and the disabled for daily care purpose, for example, wound dressings for wound caring and diapers for incontinence management. Most healthcare hygiene products that are developed are tending to be disposable products. A variety of materials are used to meet different functional performance requirements. Several reviews are presented in this chapter on the related topics of these medical healthcare products.

4.1. Superabsorbent materials (SAMs) used in disposable healthcare products

Disposable healthcare products containing superabsorbent materials (SAMs) have been used by consumers worldwide for decades. SAMs, which are made from superabsorbent polymers (SAPs), have the property of absorbing and retaining huge amount of aqueous solutions. Superabsorbent polymer materials can uptake water as high as 100,000% [229]. The absorbent hygiene products can be made thinner because smaller amount of SAPs can absorb the same volume of aqueous liquid as larger amount of fluff [230]. For this reason, they are widely adopted in the manufacturing of disposable healthcare products such as diapers, feminine care products and adult incontinence products.

SAPs are originally either natural or synthetic materials. The natural superabsorbents consist of modification of guar gum, xanthan gum or chitin, while the synthetic superabsorbents are produced by the polymerization of acrylic acid, acrylic esters, vinyl acetate, ethylene oxide, acrylamine and other vinyl monomers with subsequent cross-linking of the resultant polymer. They may be classified into three types: (1) cellulose-based SAPs; (2) starch-based SAPs; and (3) acrylamide- or acrylic acid-based synthetic SAPs [231]. Most SAPs are cross-linked copolymers of partially neutralized acrylic acid. The cross-link density and surface cross-linking of hygroscopic materials strongly affect the absorbency property of disposable hygiene products.

The polymers may be in fiber or film form, which is especially useful for absorbing body fluids [232]. Superabsorbent fibers (SAFs) can be incorporated into fabrics, yarns and absorbent products more easily. They can also be spun in blends with other fibers [233]. A superabsorbent fiber named "Lanscal F" has a fiber length of up to 51 mm. The absorbency of this fiber is up to 150 ml/g of pure water and 50 ml/g of 0.9% saline solution [234].

Antibacterial properties may be incorporated into SAFs, which contains a polymer such as polyacrylic acid and a zeolite with metal cations such as silver ions [235]. Absorbent hygiene products made of such SAF will neither give off nor develop unpleasant odor after the soaking of body fluids.

SAPs are widely applied in the medical field and personal hygiene. For example, SAPs in pads and wipes, which can rapidly immobilize large amounts of blood and other aqueous spillage, are used in operation theaters, analytical laboratories, clinics and hospitals [233].

A breathable fabric with a high resistance to penetration of aqueous liquids is developed for the making of protective garments [236].

In the application of SAM, main concern is the safety of users and carers exposed to it. Numerous studies have been done to assess the irritation and allergic potential with the application of SAMs, and no internal or external untoward/harmful effects have ever been demonstrated [237,238]. Lane et al. [239] have proved the clinical endpoints and scientific review on the safe use of three different types of cross-linked polyacrylate polymers in disposable diapers.

Another major concern is the environmental impact of disposable SAM products, and a number of studies have shown that there are no harmful effects due to soil and compost of SAMs [240–242]. Generally, SAMs are recognized as not being biodegradable because these are mostly derived from acrylic acid, which itself is derived from petroleum oil, a nonrenewable material. New development of SAMs made from biodegradable renewable resources has become necessary. New biodegradable SAMs, which are invented by Weerawarna [243], consist of composite cellulose fibers and a fiber comprising carboxyalkyl cellulose, starch and a plurality of nonpermanent intra-fiber metal cross-links.

4.2. Wound dressings

Wound dressings are materials used to cover wounds. Wounds may be caused from different mechanical injuries (e.g., abrasions, cuts, bites and invasive surgery) or burns, which may be caused by thermal, chemical, electrical and radiation injuries. Some types of chronic ulcerative wounds, which are caused from pressure sores or leg ulcers, may commonly occur among elderly people. The function of wound dressings is to provide protection to the injured wounds and safety from contamination and further injuries. The wound dressings should be easy to apply, easy to remove and able to leach toxic components.

Traditional wound dressings include various types of gauzes, such as bandages, woven, nonwoven or knitted gauzes and so on. They are often made from cotton or yarn by a simple woven technique. The appropriate wound dressing for each wound at its particular stage depends on the amount of exudates, tissue growth and healing factors. Thus, no single dressing will be suitable for use in all situations. The requirement for the wound dressing is not the same at different healing process stages and physiological conditions of wounds.

The preparation of a wound dressing mainly focuses on the balance of moisture for wound healing. If a "moist healing" condition can be created by controlling the level of moisture at the interface between the wound and the applied dressing, then it would facilitate fast wound healing, able to deal with odor, leakage, maceration and pain and prevent infection and wound deterioration [244,245]. The oxidative mechanism of iodine is broadly effective against a broad spectrum of bacteria, mycobacteria, fungi, protozoa and viruses that can be used for the prevention and treatment of infected wound. Jones and Milton [246] have studied when and how to use iodine dressings. There is a highly absorbent antimicrobial dressing suitable for excessive exudates from the wound. It is made of silver-based alginate fibers, which incorporates silver ions into alginate fibers (a natural polysaccharide extracted from brown seaweeds) [247]. Lee et al. [248], in research on dressings for malodorous wounds, have indicated that an odor-absorbent dressing with activated charcoal is the most efficient method for the absorption of unpleasant odor from infected wounds. Another antimicrobial dressing, which contains agents such as chlorhexidine, iodine or silver compounds as a barrier to the transmission of microbial pathogens, can prevent infection to the patient from external microbial pathogens [249]. The study by Rajendran [250] showed that chlorhexidine has a rapid and bactericidal activity against a wide spectrum of nonsporing bacteria. It can be widely used as an antiseptic wound dressing. Moreover, the simplicity and improvement of the electrospinning fabrication process can diversify the various applications of electrospun nanofibers in a broad range of biomedical fields and can be used as materials for wound dressing [251].

Recent new technologies have driven the development of using materials such as alginates, hydrocolloids, hydrogels and polyurethane foams for innovative wound dressing products. The design of wound dressing is also modified to shape and fit particular body contours for enhancing wound healing [252]. Although smart wound care materials are more effective and more functional than the traditional ones [253], traditional gauze materials are still used for wound dressings along with the modern high-tech dressings.

4.3. Diapers for incontinence problems

Incontinence is a problem that commonly occurs in the elderly and adults with particular illnesses. People who have difficulty in managing continence may need the support of incontinence products to contain urine leakage to maintain personal hygiene care to have a better quality of life and carry out their daily lives confidently. Diapers are the most common absorbent products that can provide healthcare hygiene support to those with an incontinence problem. Currently, diapers are available in a wide range of designs, sizes and absorbencies. Adult diapers are either disposable or reusable, and they are generally applied for moderate or heavy incontinence management [254]. In the case of light incontinence management, other incontinence products such as sanitary napkins, menstrual pads and integral pads may be used [255].

Disposable diapers generally consist of an absorbent pad sandwiched between two sheets of nonwoven fabric and their technology has continued to evolve since the 1970s [256]. Disposable diapers contain a mixture of cellulose pulp and superabsorbent polymer chemicals in the core layer that facilitate the remarkable ability to absorb up to 300 times of its weight in water [257,258]. Multilayer composites of wood pulp, synthetic fiber, binder fiber and granular superabsorbent material may also be used to achieve better fluid management and optimal absorbency for collecting fluids [259].

A diaper has a multilayer structure. The inner top layer, which is in direct contact with the skin, is made of soft polyresin fabric or nonwoven carded fiber web. This continuous filament web can provide a sense of dryness to the skin. In order to facilitate good skin care conditions, the designed pores of this microscopic funnel are large enough to let air flow in but small enough to keep water from leaking out. An acquisition layer, which would act as a blotting paper between the liner and the core, is made of synthetic fibers or modified cellulose fibers. It can allow the transfer and distribution of urine slowly and keep it locked in the core layer for reducing potential leakage. The core layer, which is made of cellulose fluff pulp combined with SAPs, can provide the absorption. The backing layer is normally a plastic film or breathable nonwoven PE film, which by using hot melt process or the heat and pressure method with direct extrusion to the film prevents wetness and dirt transfer out of the diaper [260]. The outer shell of the diaper may be covered with a layer of nonwoven material to give a cloth-like feel to the external surface.

Most diapers need to improve surface dryness and reduce tendency to leak. Therefore, the primary function of diapers is not only to increase absorbent capacity but also to immobilize fluid and prevent it from being squeezed out under pressure. The likelihood of leakage of hygiene products is related to the rate at which a fabric absorbs the liquid [261]. The absorbing capacity of a normal wood pulp is around 10 cc of water in a gram of pulp, but its capacity will drop to less than 2 cc when 5 kPa of pressure is applied [262]. An absorbent material, which comprises hydrogel-forming polymeric material and wettable staple fiber, has been developed for the improvement of liquid permeability and is good to be used as a disposable diaper [263].

The development of diapers is not only limited to the functional properties on absorbency. Many other advanced features are applied on diapers to meet various requirements. For example, special sizing and coloring are designed for specific gender and age, and a color-change indicator is added to provide a wet signal when the diaper is to be changed [264]. Adjustable belted diaper [265,276] is designed with an adjustable and reattachable Velcro-type closure or pull-up design diaper [267] that facilitates an easier way for the frail elderly with incontinence or the disabled to dress themselves.

Fader et al. [268] have made comparisons of absorbent incontinence products of various designs. Their findings showed that a pull-up diaper was overall better than other designs as it was easier to apply and quicker to change, but was more expensive. A T-shaped diaper was not better than the traditional disposable one. Combination uses of different designed products might be involved for cost-effective management during daytime or nighttime and in different circumstances within a limited budget. The users might use more effective and expensively designed diapers when going out. On the contrary, they might use less effective and cheaply designed diapers when staying at home.

5. Review of intelligent medical garments

Smart or intelligent clothing is a garment with sensing and actuation properties that is able to sense external stimuli and respond with active control to those stimuli. The first generation of intelligent garments is developed by fitting electronic components and conventional materials into daily clothing [269]. The innovation of smart or intelligent textiles, new sensors, miniaturization, computing science and related technologies in recent years has enabled the development of intelligent clothing in the biomedical and healthcare fields. The intelligent medical garment, which is made by the integration of microelectronics and smart textiles, is generally used to collect physiological and/or biological data and provide risk assessment, diagnosis and function as health monitoring for particular cases or individual needs.

Axisa et al. [270] divided smart clothing into two groups:

- Smart clothing with sensors located in proximity to the skin. Sensing fabrics [271,272] can be used to make a smart garment with sensors, which are embedded in the layers of fabric or on fabric surface.
- Smart clothing involves the use of intelligent devices, which are simply placed in a pocket of the garment.

As the sensors or sensing system of intelligent medical garment is located precisely into the garment in a discreet, nonvisible and well-protected way, an intelligent medical garment is user-friendly and well adapted for monitoring chronic diseases of the disabled and the elderly.

5.1. Application of conductive textile material into the smart garment

Conductive textile material is an integral part of a smart garment. Textile materials can be made conductive by many methods, which may include manufacturing of fabric with conductive yarns/fibers, nonconducting fabric coated with conductive material or engrafting of metallic fibers/particles in the textile fibers. All materials with properties of high electric conductivity can be used as conductive fibers. The conductive yarns are usually coated with polyester or polyamide and a thin layer of silver in order to improve corrosion resistance as well as to be insulated from exposure to humid environments. Silver-plated copper wire was considered as the most suitable material for conductive fibers to enhance power and signal transmissions [273].

For integration of conductive materials into daily clothing, it should be functional, lightweight, flexible and durable. A type of lightweight hybrid metal–polymer yarn, which has a lower electrical conductivity than copper, was developed as an alternative to heavy copper wiring [274]. The integration of this hybrid metal–polymer material in textiles makes production of truly flexible, soft, lightweight and comfortable smart clothing possible. Unlike conventional rigid electronic components, the soft touch switching technology with wearable interaction interfaces, which can be incorporated into textiles or sewn on daily clothing, has also been developed [275].

By means of the tubular intarsia technique, Paradiso et al. [276,277] developed fabric electrodes, which are made of metal-based conductive yarns and are knitted in a multilayered structure. The conductive surface is sandwiched between the insulated textile surfaces, and contact between metal and skin only exists in the electrode regions. The study by Pacelli et al. [278] showed that conductive fabric electrodes applied on fabrics could be used for monitoring physiological and biomechanical variables. Piezo-resistive yarns, optic fibers and color multilayers can be used as sensors in garments [279]. By integrating electronic components, phase change materials, shape memory materials or nanomaterials, various smart garments can be designed with special properties involving mechanical, chemical, electrical and thermal performances [280] in the health industry.

5.2. Examples of intelligent medical garments

Basically, intelligent medical garments are developed on the basis of the full integration of sensors, actuators, energy sources and information processing and communication functions of e-textiles. These could be worn comfortably all day long and made operational continuously without restriction on their mobility and without hindrance to the wearers' daily activities. Most intelligent medical garments are designed with a wearable health monitoring system. It ranges from a jacket, vest, diapers and even outfit accessories such as on-wrist device or belt-worn PCs.

5.2.1. Smart garments for vital signs and motion monitoring

Intelligent medical garments can be used to record biological signals of physiological states for the daily health monitoring of wearers or even provide real-time feedback to medical or nursing personnel for appropriate treatment. There are various types of wearable healthcare devices. Some of them involve the use of sensors and medical devices simply housed in the pockets of the general daily garments. Others are wearable vital or motion monitoring garments, which are capable to measure specific vital signs, including heart rate, respiratory rate, oxygen saturation, body temperature as well as detecting falls and location of the elderly wearer. These medical garments offer a powerful new way not only to keep track of the ailing patients' medical conditions and predict impending events but also to help healthy users to monitor their physiological states while performing high-risk activities or during exercise training [281]. Some of these medical devices/garments are discussed as follows:

- The Georgia Tech wearable motherboard (GTWM) is probably the first intelligent medical garment. It uses an electrical wiring system with conventional sensors to measure different physiological parameters, including heart rate (electrocardiogram, ECG), respiratory rate and body temperature [282]. This intelligent medical garment is woven as an undershirt design and various fiber materials could be applied for a specific functionality [283]. For example, Spandex is used for better elasticity and good fitting; Nega-Stat is used for better antistatic properties and optical fibers are used to detect bullet wounds.

- On the basis of the "wearable motherboard" technology from Georgia Tech, Sensatex developed "SmartShirt" [284], which is a unisex wearable T-shirt made of cotton fabric integrated with conductive fibers to set up a connective system for collecting physiological signals, including heart rate, respiration rate, body temperature and blood pressure of the wearer [285]. The collected data are digitized and sent either by Bluetooth or ZigBee wireless technology to a remote base station for data monitoring [286,287].

- The system of Advanced Medical Monitor (AMON) is worn on the wrist as a watch-like unit [288]. It is composed of sensors, communication and processing devices, which are capable of collecting and evaluating multiple medical parameters, including heart rate, heart rhythm, oxygen saturation (SpO_2) and skin temperature. The device can also monitor the activities and mobility of the wearer via acceleration sensors for detecting potentially dangerous falls [289]. Extra sensors can optionally be installed for monitoring physiological data, such as ECG, electroencephalogram (EEG), serum glucose level and respiratory peak-flow [270].

- A textile-based wearable system, named MagIC (Maglietta Interattiva Computerizzata), is composed of a vest or a jacket with textile sensors woven into the garment through a computer-aided design/computer-aided manufacture (CAD/CAM) process at the thorax level to obtain an ECG lead and respiratory rate, and a portable electronic board, which is placed on the garment by a Velcro strip for detecting ECG, respiratory signals and the wearer's motion [290–292]. This vital vest or jacket is made of cotton and Lycra. The elastic properties of these fabrics can guarantee that the electrodes on the garment have a good contact with the wearer's body. Different sensors can be integrated into the garment for collecting various physiological parameters of vital signs, including ECG, EEG, electromyogram (EMG), diastolic and systolic blood pressure, heart rate, respiratory frequency, body temperature, serum glucose level and so on. All collected physiological data from the sensors are transmitted automatically via a wireless Bluetooth connection to a remote computer and to the patient's cell phone or personal digital assistant (PDA) for data visualization and storage on disk or memory card in order to provide multi-sources and real-time physiological data to doctors. The data or alarm is sent to the central alarm system to notify the healthcare providers if any abnormal medical situation is detected [293].

- VivoMetrics has developed a "LifeShirt," which uses embedded sensors woven into the shirt to associate with a PDA to set up a multifunction and ambulatory system for monitoring and recording more than 30 vital signs data of the wearer, including ECG, respiratory monitoring, heart function, apnea detection, posture and physical activity level and so on [294,295]. The collected data are uploaded onto a computer and sent back to the monitoring center via Internet. Then, the data are analyzed and sent back to the wearer and the clinicians for a better understanding of the wearer's health [296].

- A medical tele-assistance suit was developed in the VTAMN project [297] ("Vêtement de Télé Assistance Médicale Nomade", which means "Underclothes for ambulatory Medical Tele Assistance"), with the aim of telemonitoring patients at risk [298]. The overall system of this medical garment incorporates four smooth dry ECG electrodes, a respiratory rate sensor, two temperature sensors with electronics, a shock/fall detection sensor and global system for mobile communication/global positioning system (GSM/GPS) modules [299]. This medical suit with integrated sensors could help to reduce medical follow-up of patients who are medically dependent.
- Intelligent medical garments for fall detection and mobile monitoring can be designed on the basis of the use of accelerometers as the sensors to measure acceleration of the wearer. Accelerometers can be mounted on different limbs or on the body trunk to measure motion and collect the accelerometer signals [300]. The Complete Ambient Assisted Living Experiment (CAALYX) system has been developed as a "Fall and Mobility Monitoring Vest" for detecting falls of the elderly [301]. The collected information from the wearable device with tri-axial accelerometers can be communicated in real time with a healthcare and emergency service provider either via PC with a broadband connection in-house or through a smart phone using a Bluetooth connection outdoors [302,303].
- A loose-fitting comfortable monitoring medical garment named SMASH was developed for posture and movement rehabilitation. Acceleration sensors are distributed and integrated into a loose-fitting long sleeved shirt as a comfortable monitoring garment to provide postural resolution of wearer's movement [304]. All data collected from this sensing garment are sent to an outer PC or an integrated Bluetooth module for offline analysis. In the study, Harms et al. [305] showed that the performance of loose-fitting SMASH was almost the same as tight-fitting sensing garment.

Table 1 lists the above-mentioned smart garments in healthcare.

5.2.2. Smart diapers

The development of smart diapers for detecting wetness provides great benefits for ailing patients who are unable to replace diapers by themselves in particular, or for those who are unable to notify their carers about wetting of diapers. Smart diapers consist of a moisture detection system, which is incorporated into traditional diapers. When the degree of wetness

Table 1. Summary of examples of an intelligent medical garment.

Example	Clothing types	Vital signs monitoring	Posture motion monitoring
GTWM	Undershirt	✓	
SmartShirt	T-shirt	✓	
AMON	Wrist-worn unit	✓	
MagIC	Vest or jacket	✓	
LifeShirt	Vest	✓	
VTAMN	T-shirt	✓	✓
CAALYX	Wearable unit or vest	✓	✓
SMASH	Loose-fitting long sleeve shirt		✓

has exceeded a predetermined threshold limit, the system sounds an alarm or sends a signal to a computer, informing the carer that the diaper of the wearer needs to be changed. The use of smart diapers in hospitals and elderly care units is not only able to decrease carers' workloads but also improves the quality of care service for the patients and avoids disturbance of checking diapers, especially during nighttime.

Sidén et al. [306] developed a paper-based, disposable, moisture-activated radio frequency identification technology (RFID) system [307], which could be incorporated into traditional cellulose-based diapers. The wireless moisture-activated sensor would emit an RF signal upon moisture detection. The handheld signal receiver detects and receives signals back from the tags. A receive-signal reader unit with an external antenna could be mounted around the ward. As the signal is detected, an alarm, such as audio buzz and blinking light, is produced on the alert line of the standard ward system to notify the carer to change a patients soiled diaper.

Yambem et al. [308] developed a wireless sensor system, which is composed of an interrogator antenna and a passive LC-resonator sensor tag for smart diaper application. The wireless inductive link between the interrogator antenna and the sensor tag is achieved through RF inductive coupling. Any change in the resonant frequency of the sensor tag will significantly modify the inductive link, which will be reflected back into the interrogator circuit and trigger an "ON/OFF" signal. This wireless sensor system is suitable for smart diaper application to detect whether the diaper is in "wet" or "dry" condition.

Another attempt, a flexible surface wetness sensor and its detected signals transmitted using the RFID technique, was developed by Yang et al. [309]. Such flexible sensor consists of an RF identification integrated circuit (RFIC) and a sensor circuit, which contains a comb-shaped sensing area surrounded by an octagonal antenna. The detected signals of wet/dry surface are transmitted through RF waves from the RFIC to a remote reader located within 15 cm. The reader of such a system might be located under or near the patient's bed. However, carer might forget to change the battery of the reader after a certain period. Handheld receivers can be integrated into this system to widen the sensitivity range of receiving the signal up to 1–1.5 m. Moreover, the Bluetooth technology can also be employed to extend the transmitting range up to 3 m from the reader to the host.

Although there are many types of moisture detecting systems available for smart diapers, there are still some significant problems with the existing wetness sensors and monitoring systems that have to be solved, that is, the sensors are not reusable and they do not gather actual wetness data directly. The wetness measurement from the diapers contains large quantities of information pertaining to the wearer's health condition, which could be useful to the medical or nursing staff in providing appropriate care and treatment to the wearer.

6. Case studies in the development of apparel for the elderly and the disabled

In the development of apparel for the elderly and the disabled, basically, the following three main techniques could be applied:

- *The selection of appropriate material*: Clothing must always be made from the finest and most appropriate materials, which includes the shell fabric and fastenings. The factors that determine the selection of material include appearance, comfort, durability and safety. Most important, the properties of material to meet the functional requirements of medical clothing cannot be excluded from consideration. The hand-feel and sensation that the material imparts would have a great effect on garment comfort. Therefore, heavy, stiff and rough materials are uncomfortable for medical garments or apparel for the elderly and the disabled, as they may cause skin irritation.

As each type of material has its own properties, it is not unusual that medical garments or apparel for the elderly and the disabled are made of a combination of different materials to provide best of quality.

- *Alteration of the pattern drafting*: Body changes, such as decreasing heights, lowering of bust lines, developing rounded backs, abdominal extensions and so on, commonly take place in most of the elderly. People with a disability also have problems with changing figure proportions. Due to physical changes in the body of the elderly and the disabled, their body measurements may differ substantially from the standard body sizes, and their body figures may also not be of the right proportions or are asymmetrical. Size and fit play an important role in the comfort of the garment. If the elderly and the disabled wear garments made under normal pattern drafting techniques, no matter how good the quality of the material for making of the garment, the wearer would still feel uncomfortable because of the poor garment fittings or poor aesthetic appearance. Thus, alteration of pattern drafting becomes necessary to alleviate the fitting problems and to improve garment comfort and appearance. The principle of ergonomics is to be applied in the pattern drafting, particularly for the elderly and the disabled clothing.
- *Modification of the clothing design*: The physical condition of the elderly and the disabled may cause difficulties in putting on and taking off the garment, or may affect their outlook image. By modifying the design of the clothing, the garment would be easy to put on and take off, and would complement the complexion and disability of the individual. Clothing designed for the elderly and the disabled could also be visually good-looking and must be suited to the person wearing it. Most important of all, the garments would not look noticeably different from the clothes that able-bodied people usually wear. Modifications in the design of medical clothing or apparel for the elderly and the disabled are needed to camouflage their figure faults or individual irregularities. The problem of the wearer would no longer be noticed if the clothing design could successfully draw the attention away from the parts that the wearer wants to conceal.

Four cases in the development of apparel for the elderly and the disabled are selected to demonstrate how these techniques are applied in the development of such apparel products.

6.1. Stoma bag underpants

For their patients having a surgical treatment on colon, such as the removal of distal sigmoid and rectum, the open end of the remaining intestine will be pulled through the abdominal wall and attached to the skin. Doctors will cut an opening called stoma on the abdomen of the patient. This enables a stoma bag to be directly connected to the intestine. The body discharge can then flow out into the stoma bag instead of flowing down into the body discharge organs.

6.1.1. Existing problems faced by the users carrying stoma bag

When a stoma bag is hung at the surface of the abdomen, the user feels uncomfortable for the extra loading of a filled stoma bag. Some users are worried that the stoma bag may not be attached properly at an appropriate position, while some users feel embarrassed when the stoma bag is seen by others when changing the clothes. The location of the stoma is usually at the left or right side of the umbilicus. To avoid contact pressure on the surface of the stoma bag, many users wear their underpants below the stoma, as shown in Figure 1. In some cases, users have complaints on wearing underpants at such a low waist level. They

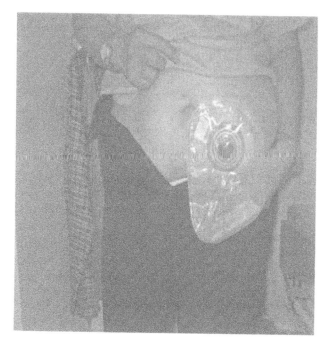

Figure 1. Stoma bag hung at the surface of the abdomen.

would feel more comfortable to wear underpants at normal waistline. Some users also have physiological discomfort to see their body discharge in stoma bag.

6.1.2. Techniques adopted for the development of stoma bag underpants

Modifications are made to the design of conventional underpants. Stoma bag underpants are designed with a pouch, which can provide support and conceal the stoma bag. An opening is made on the underpants, which matches the size and location of the stoma on the abdomen, as shown in Figure 2. It enables the underpants to be worn at the normal waistline. As the stoma bag will be hung on the surface of the underpants instead of being placed underneath, it is more comfortable for the patients. A zip opening may be added on the pouch, which allows the user or carer to check the stoma bag easily without taking off the underpants.

6.2. Urine bag pants

Incontinence is a common problem associated with bladder and kidney malfunctioning. Many persons who suffer from urology problems and incontinence may need to carry a urine bag for collecting urine through urethra. Such a system for collecting urine discharge comprises a long catheter and a plastic bag big enough to hold a considerable amount of urine (usually from 500 to 1000 cc). The urine bag is required to be emptied when it is filled by urine. This is performed through the readily accessible valve on the urine bag. When urinary catheter is used, it is inserted into the urethra of the patient and is taken out and reset only for medical examination or treatment.

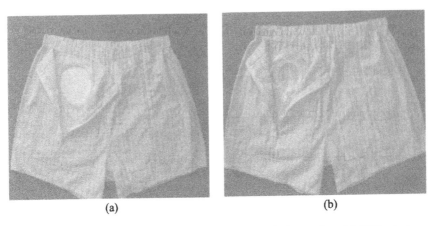

(a)   (b)

Figure 2. Stoma bag underpants designed with a pouch and zip opening. (a) Without stoma bag inside the pouch; (b) with stoma bag inside the pouch.

6.2.1. *Problems faced by people carrying a urine bag*

Most patients who use a urine bag do not like its unusual appearance. Having to carry it hurts their confidence and self-esteem. Most people prefer to conceal the urine bag in the best way. For example, the urine bag is hung on their waist and covered up by an overcoat as shown in Figure 3. As the urine bag has to be hung at or below the level of the urethra, the length of the overcoat should be long enough to cover it. This is inconvenient for the wearer in hot and humid environments. It is also very common to tie the urine bag on the leg of the wearer and cover it with pants. The tightness of leg straps around the lower extremity can cause irritation to skin or even constriction to the circulation to the lower portion of leg

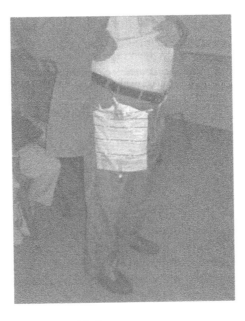

Figure 3. Urine bag hung on waist outside the trousers.

S.-F. Ng et al.

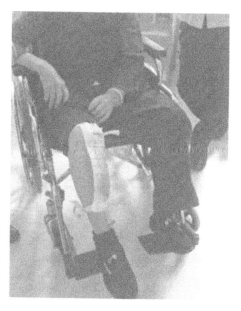

Figure 4.   Urine bag tied on the leg of the patient covered with trousers.

as shown in Figure 4. In particular, it is uncomfortable to have a strap wrapped around the leg for long hours every day. Some people attempt to conceal the urine bag by just putting it inside a bag as shown in Figure 5, but the tube of the urine bag still remains uncovered and the urine bag is recognized easily.

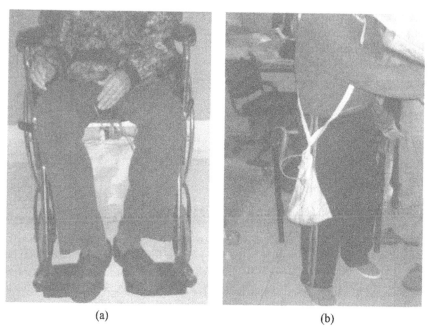

(a)   (b)

Figure 5.   The urine bag used by the patient is concealed by a plastic or cloth bag.

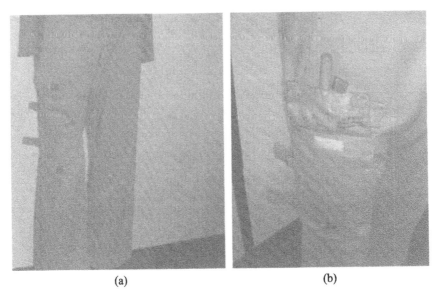

(a)   (b)

Figure 6.   The urine bag used by the patient can be concealed in the pocket of the pants.

6.2.2. Techniques adopted for the development of urine bag pants

The urine bag could be camouflaged by inserting it into a special pocket of urine bag pants, which makes the wearer happier because they are not exposing it to the public. Instead of using a conventional patch pocket to hold the urine bag, the urine bag pocket is specially designed to adapt to the requirements for camouflaging it, as shown in Figure 6. It possesses an opening on the back for inverting the urine bag. The catheter, which is linked with the penis or bladder of the user, can be directed along a channel on the inside of pants and be directed to the back of the pocket. The specially designed pocket also possesses a lower opening, which is the outlet of the discharge valve of the urine bag. Without such lower opening on the pocket, the urine bag has to be taken out from the pocket whenever it is to be emptied, and the discharge valve would be bent inside the pocket, which causes a higher risk of urine leakage. There is also a downward flap for concealing the discharge valve that helps to further camouflage the urine bag while still allowing easy access to the discharge valve. The adaptive design of the pocket on urine bag pants helps incontinence sufferers to maintain dignity as their urine bag is fully camouflaged without affecting their movements or mobility.

6.3. Pants for chair-bound people

People who are physically disabled either due to chronic sickness or aging spend a great part of each day in a seated position or confined to wheelchairs. The sedentary body may have physical changes, which makes it different to the body of an ambulatory person. When the elderly or the disabled remain in a seating posture for a long period, the spine curves forward and stretches the garment from the waistline to the collar at the back. The waistline of the pants will be pulled and dropped at the back, and the length from the waistline to the front crotch would be reduced. In addition, the body tends to spread in girth, particularly at thighs and buttocks. Thus, their pants tend to tighten around the thighs and the crotch can be cut into skin.

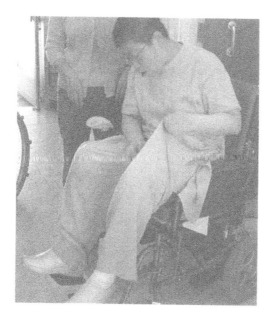

Figure 7. The common problem encountered by chair-bound people.

6.3.1. Problems faced by chair-bound people

Conventional pants are designed for an ambulatory person based on a standing position. The problems encountered by a chair-bound person who needs pants designed for a seated figure are not considered, as shown in Figure 7. When the wearer who is permanently sedentary puts on a pair of conventional pants that is made under standard measurements, the waistline of the pants will be slant from the front to the back of the body. The pulling of fabric at the back rise seam and the bunching of fabric at the front rise seam are common occurrences. Such poor garment fitting will cause discomfort, more so when a person is seated for long periods. The extra material in the lower abdominal area and at the upper portion of the leg would create creases and unpleasant bulges of fabric, which would affect the wearer's image and self-esteem.

When the wearer is seated and the legs are bent, the pants tend to ride up on the leg. This will cause the hosiery or bare legs being exposed, as pants length will look shorter. Conversely, due to the measurement taken over the bent knee, the length from hip to ankle would increase. A common problem encountered by chair-bound people is the hem of pants looks longer at the back and shorter at the front. This is opposite to the conventional pattern cutting of standard pants, which are normally cut with the hemline slightly longer at the back than at the front. Such inappropriate pattern cutting of pants would affect the appearance of the wearer

6.3.2. Techniques applied for the development of pants for chair-bound people

Special thought should be given to the pants that are designed for the elderly or the disabled who are chair-bound. In order to improve the comfort and appearance of the pants, following alterations (as shown in Figure 8) on pattern drafting should be made to accommodate the requirements of a seated figure and also provide a greater ease of movement.

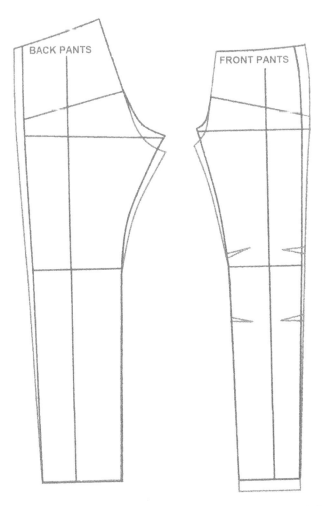

Figure 8. Application of pattern alternation to improve fittings of the pants for chair-bound people.

- In order to maintain the waistline of pants at the same level from the floor, and to remove the extra fabric folds across the abdominal area when the person is in a seated posture, the pattern of the pants should be adjusted to make the waistline higher at the back and lower at the front when compared with the conventional fitting pants.
- The hemline of the flat pattern needs to be adjusted by taking out the excess fabric at the back and increasing the length at the front for balancing the problem that pants tend to ride up on the leg when the wearer is seated and the legs are bent. In some cases, a small tuck or dart can be added behind the knee to provide better fitting for bent legs.
- Due to the change of the body girth in the abdominal, thighs and buttock areas, extra room should be designed into pants for chair-bound people. Ease should be increased at the back pieces by reshaping the back rise and side seams.

Apart from the application of pattern alteration to improve the fitting of the pants for chair-bound people, the pants may also modify the design into an elasticated waistline on back. Such a design would make the waistband more adjustable and can provide better comfort. The fabric material selected for making the pants is also important. Knitted fabric with good stretchability would help in providing better comfort and fit to the chair-bound people.

6.4. Sun block protective garments for patients with xeroderma pigmentosum

Xeroderma pigmentosum (XP) is a rare hereditary disease related to DNA pathology, which causes abnormalities in eye and skin pigmentation. The DNA damage is cumulative and irreversible, and there is no cure for XP. The victim of such disease is extremely allergic to ultraviolet (UV) rays. Even minimal exposure to UV rays can result into acute sunburn reaction and skin lesions.

6.4.1. Problems faced by patients with XP

People suffering from XP have to avoid all sources of UV radiation. Various preventive measures, such as taking an umbrella for all outdoor activities (as shown in Figure 9), are introduced to protect the body surfaces of such patients from UV radiation, but it is quite inconvenient for the patients to bring along the umbrella all the time. This measure is still inadequate to provide complete UV protection due to the presence of an unnoticeable source of UV exposure in living environment. Applying high sun protective factor (SPF) sunscreen to face and all exposed body parts is another common method, as shown in Figure 10. However, it is difficult to ensure that the application of a sunblock lotion could cover every small area of the exposed skin, and this needs constant reapplication at regular intervals, or it will wear away or wash off.

If people suffering from XP need to engage in outdoor activities during the daytime, they would put on long sleeved jackets, long pants, gloves and sunglasses. To protect their face and neck, a face mask or a head-cover, which looks like a helmet, is commonly used for UV protection. The head-cover is made of a transparent plastic sheet, which is a UV protective material. It covers the whole face and neck without blocking the vision. Even though the head-cover is effective for protection, the wearer feels embarrassed by its

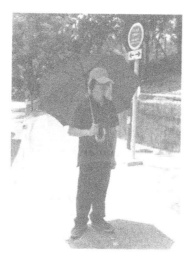

Figure 9. XP sufferer carrying an umbrella for UV protection.

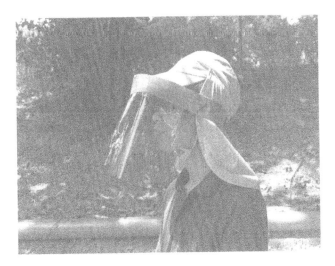

Figure 10. XP sufferer wearing a helmet for UV protection.

unpleasant appearance and is reluctant to put it on among peer groups. Due to the lack of an appropriate protective garment, some patients try to avoid or reduce their outdoor activities.

6.4.2. Techniques applied for the development of a sunblock protective garment for patients with XP

Clothing can provide an effective barrier to UV radiation, but careful selection of fabric is important to achieve sufficient ultraviolet protection factor (UPF) and SPF. Although all fabrics can offer sun protection to some extent, the fabrics that protect well against UV rays are generally tight weaves and with chemical sunscreens added. A fabric's SPF would increase with an increase in mass or weight. Dark color fabrics provide increased protection compared with white color fabrics. Unlike the sun protective clothing, which is designed for people on leisure such as on the beach, the fabric used for sunblock protective clothing designed for patients of XP needs better durability, as it would be used daily by them.

In order to solve the above-stated problem, the design of a conventional jacket could be modified with the following special features, as shown in Figure 11:

- A hood is needed to cover the neck and head of the patient. An enlarged rim is added along the edge of the hood to shield the face from sunlight.
- The collar is designed as a facemask, which could cover the portion of face below the eyes. The whole face of the wearer could be covered by the hood and collar with the addition of a pair of sunglasses. The collar can be opened at the center front and turned down as a conventional convertible collar.
- The length of the sleeve is designed with extra length and elasticated cuff, which enables it to cover the upper limbs, including the fingers. The elasticated cuff permits the wearer to pull the sleeve up to wrist level and down to cover the whole hand and fingers without any difficulty.

Apart from the assurance of UV protection, the design of this sunblock protective garment is intended to provide a more dignified and normalized look to the wearer. This is important to the wearer in their social life.

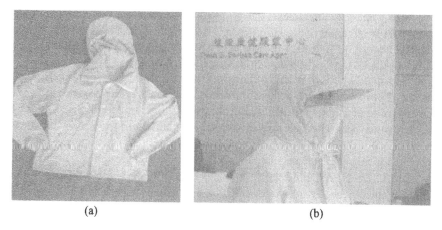

(a)   (b)

Figure 11.   New design of UV protective clothing.

7. Future prospects of developing apparel for the elderly and the disabled

A higher quality of life is now expected by the elderly and the disabled. As clothes remain in direct contact with the skin of the elderly and the disabled, the improvement of quality and efficiency of medical garments and apparel for the elderly and the disabled has become more important. Due to increasing shortage of HCWs in hospitals, nursing homes and in home care, it is necessary for the development of new healthcare apparel products to reduce the workloads of carers and to provide a great care toward the elderly and the disabled. For ailing patients who are unable to replace wet diapers by themselves, the advent of smart diapers makes it possible to detect wetness and inform carers to change it at a proper time. Several sensor systems have been developed for smart diaper applications; for example, Siden et al. [310] developed a paper-based disposable moisture-activated RFID system that could be incorporated into the traditional cellulose-based diaper. Lamyanba Yambem et al. [308] developed a low-cost wireless sensor system for smart diaper, but it only detects whether the diaper is in a "wet" or "dry" condition. The other attempt is a flexible surface wetness sensor using RFID technique developed by Yang et al. [311]. Their sensor system is able to detect the radio signal by a reader in the range of 15 cm. The reader of this system might be located under or near the patient's bed, and the sensitivity range of receiving the signal is restricted to about 1–1.5 m. A significant problem with the existing wetness sensors and monitoring systems used on smart diapers is that the sensors are not reusable and do not gather actual wetness data, which could be useful to reflect the wearer's health condition.

There is a great demand for the development of eco-friendly reusable diapers. Obviously, the use of disposable smart diapers with electronic systems is uneconomical and hazardous to the environment, but there are possibilities to develop a nondisposable remote wetness detection system for smart diapers before a complete reusable smart diaper comes out. A new smart diaper could also be used to collect actual wetness data, which may pertain to the wearer's health conditions. In the case of bladder control training, which is given to incontinence patients, a therapist can monitor the progress of the bladder training if the data collected from smart diapers show the quantity and frequency of wetness per day. In addition, the wetting detection system may integrate with other detection systems. For example, an alarm or signal may be sent to a caretaker when the wearer of a smart diaper moves beyond a predetermined threshold limit. There have been many developments in the field of intelligent medical garments that are used for health monitoring. Most of them are composed of various types of detecting sensors. Improvements can be made by reducing the size and number of the detecting sensors, and it would be ideal if multifunctional sensors could be developed for the detection or measurement of vital signs.

The frail elderly have problems of cognitive weakness, weakened muscles, joints and ligaments. They may also have medical problems concurrently with hindrance in movement after illness or traumatic injury such as a stroke, spinal cord injury, orthopedic surgery and so on. They would need a beneficial rehabilitation program to assist them to restore their lost function caused by their weakened extremities and disability. In particular, for the group of geriatric and amputee patients who have difficulties in understanding new information, following commands and doing rehab activities effectively, the development of medical clothing with electric assistive devices can play a significant role in helping the elderly or the disabled to have control over their body functions and abilities. For example, a robotic exoskeleton suit named hybrid assistive limb (HAL) can provide human-like movement to the wearer. The application of this medical clothing can assist in walking and performing daily routine activities in cases of stroke-induced paralysis or spinal cord injury patients and the frail elderly [312]. There are sensors on the power suit, which can detect the nerve signals on the skin surface. The detected nerve signals are sent from the brain to the particular muscles for movement. The power suit could interpret the planned movement, assist to move in unison with the wearer's limbs, augment human motion and reinforce the strength before the muscles actually work. If no bioelectrical signals are detected, the suit can also provide human-like movement based on the stored information. Another power robotic jacket, which can help hemiplegic and post-stroke patients recover from partial paralysis during rehabilitation, was also developed by Matsushita Electric Industrial. There are artificial muscles on the paralyzed side powered by compressed air and controlled by four sensors, which are attached to the elbow and wrist of the healthy arm. The sensors can sense the muscle contraction of the healthy side and control the artificial muscles of the paralyzed side simultaneously in order to optimize muscle strengthening therapy [313].

The application of robotic clothing for rehabilitation is beneficial to patients and the elderly, but the weight of the existing robotic clothing still is a burden for the wearer, in particular for the frail elderly or disabled patients. Further studies should be concentrated on the amelioration of textiles and materials for manufacturing this robot jacket to make it lighter in weight. It will then be easier for the disabled wearer to use it independently.

The use of textiles patches for delivering of drugs has already been explored by the pharmaceutical industry. There has been a trend to develop medical clothing for clinical treatment. Microencapsulation technology is one of the effective techniques toward the development of new medical textiles for cosmetic or clinical purposes. Microencapsulation technology is actually a micro-packaging technique involving the production of micro-capsules, and it is also known as micro-particles containing some kind of chemicals or extracts. The micro-capsules could be grafted into textile materials for the development of novel textiles. Gelatine/vitamin C has been successfully grafted into fibrous material by using the emulsion hardening technique with formaldehyde as a cross-linking agent. Vitamin C will be released from the gelatine wall shell in the presence of humidity due to its sensitivity to moisture and hence absorbed directly by the human skin [314]. A new attempt is to use traditional Chinese herbal medicine for the treatment of AD by means of medical clothing. In the treatment of AD, using traditional Chinese medicine as an alternative systemic therapy is increasingly popular and it can be administered in oral, topical and photo-chemotherapeutic modalities, as well as in injectable forms [315]. The integration of using an effective traditional Chinese medicine formula as a systemic therapy for AD with textile materials by microencapsulation technology would be a new possibility for the development of novel medical textiles. The prospects for developing biomedical textiles for manufacturing medical garments or apparel for the elderly and the disabled are numerous. The concept of integrating microcapsulation or nanocapsulation technology with medicine can be further transferred to other medical diseases. Although the use of medical garments for the treatment of diseases is still not fully explored, their development would grow at a cruise speed by intense cooperation between people from various disciplines, including textile scientists, bioengineers, medical professionals and fashion designers. It is not only the development of novel smart textiles that is important for the future development of medical garments or clothing for the elderly and the disabled: the comfort, durability and aesthetic value are also crucial for the overall quality of medical garments.

8. Conclusion

There is no doubt that the use of smart textiles will be able to apply to medical clothing and apparel for the elderly and the disabled. The development of smart garments for the healthcare industry is the next frontier of convergence of different technologies for clinical or rehabilitation purposes. However, clothing is a basic need of all people. The application of medical garments and apparel for the elderly and the disabled should be interpreted in a broad sense. Apart from high-tech clothing designed for specific functions, casual clothing is also important for the elderly and the disabled. The application of medical garments and apparel for the elderly and the disabled in the long term should be widened to more daily applications. Appropriately designed medical garments and apparel for the elderly and the disabled not only help the wearer in the aspects of protection, caring or medical treatment but also provide enhancement of their personal capabilities and quality of life. Thus, the medical value, symbolic value and the comfort factor are the main concerns in the development of these apparel products in the healthcare industry.

References

[1] A. Mathews and M. Hardingham, *Medical and Hygiene Textile Production: A Handbook*, Intermediate Technology, London, 1994.
[2] A.J. Rigby and S.C. Anand, *Medical textiles*, in *Handbook of Technical Textiles*, Chap. 15, A.R. Horrocks and S.C. Anand, eds., CRC Press, Boca Raton, FL, 2000, pp. 407–424. Available at http://www.knovel.com/web/portal/basic_search/display?_EXT_KNOVEL_DISPLAY_bookid=926 (accessed Feb 2011).
[3] S. Rajendran and S.C. Anand, Text. Intell. 2nd Quarter (2001) p. 25.
[4] S. Rajendran and S.C. Anand, Text. Prog. 32(4) (2002), Textile Institute Manchester, UK.
[5] M. Tatsuki, Text. Prog. 40(3) (2008, Sep) pp. 123–181. Available at http://www.informaworld.com/smpp/section?content=a903103085&fulltext=713240928 (accessed Oct 2009).
[6] M. Thoren, *A new approach to clothing for disabled users*, Chap. 14, in *Perspectives in Rehabilitation Ergonomics*, K. Shrawan, ed., Taylor & Francis, London, 1997, p. 360.
[7] B. Le Pechoux and T.K. Ghosh, Text. Prog. 32(1) (2002) Textile Institute, Manchester, UK.
[8] A. Sabit, *Wellington Sears Handbook of Industrial Textiles*, Technomic, Lancaster, PA, 1995.
[9] J.W.S. Hearle, *Fibres and fabrics for protective textiles*, in *Textiles for Protection*, R.A. Scott ed., CRC Press, Boca Raton, FL, 2005, pp. 117–150.
[10] C. Byrne, *Technical textiles market – an overview*, in *Handbook of Technical Textiles*, A.R. Horrocks and S.C. Anand eds., Woodhead, Cambridge, 2000, pp. 1–23.
[11] W. Zhou, N. Reddy and Y. Yang, *Overview of protective clothing*, in *Textiles for Protection*, R.A. Scott ed., CRC Press, Boca Raton, FL, 2005, pp. 3–30.
[12] US Department of Labor – Occupational Safety and Health Administration (OSHA), *Gowns, Aprons, and Other Protective Body Clothing*, 1910.1030(d)(3)(xi). Available at http://

www.osha.gov/pls/oshaweb/owadisp.show_document?p_table=standards&p_id=10051 (accessed Aug 2010).

[13] R.A. Scott, *Textiles for Protection,* CRC Press, Boca Raton, FL, 2005.

[14] W. Whyte, P.V. Bailey, D.L. Hamblen, W.D. Fisher and I.G. Kelly, J. Bone Joint Surg. Br. 65(4) (1983, Aug), pp. 502–506.

[15] J.A. Moylan, K.T. Fitzpatrick and K.E. Davenport, Arch. Surg. 122(2) (1987, Feb), pp. 152–157.

[16] Health Care Industry, AORN J. (2003, Jan). Available at http://findarticles.com/p/articles/mi_m0FSL/is_1_77/ai_97058878/pg_2/ (accessed Aug 2010).

[17] J.R. Wagner and H.A. Hager, Tappi. J. 80(9) (1997) pp. 167–172.

[18] P.M. Avinash, Text. Res. J. 78(8) (2008, Aug) pp. 710–717.

[19] L. Van Langenhove, R. Puers and D. Matthys, *Intelligent textiles for medical applications: an overview,* in *Medical Textiles And Biomaterials For Healthcare, Incorporating, Proceedings of International Conference and Exhibition on Healthcare and Medical Textiles, 2003, The University of Bolton,* Woodhead, Cambridge, 2006.

[20] The Free Library.com, *Hospital/medical applications: For polyolefin nonwoven products.* Available at http://www.thefreelibrary.com/Hospital%2fmedical+applications%3a+for+polyolefin+nonwoven+products.-a08167597 (accessed Aug 2010).

[21] C.D. Goad and J.L. Taylor, *Woven medical fabric,* Precision Fabrics Group, Greensboro, NC; Standard Textile Co., Inc., Cincinnati, OH. US Patent 4822667, 18 April, 1989.

[22] DuPont, *Tyvek for aprons, gowns & smocks.* Available at http://www2.dupont.com/Personal_Protection/en_US/products/controlled_env/garment_styles/aprons_gowns_smocks.html (accessed Aug 2010).

[23] R.R. Mather, *Polyolefin fibres – healthcare and medical applications,* Chap. 5, in *Synthetic Fibres: Nylon, Polyester, Acrylic, Polyolefin,* J.E. McIntyre, ed., CRC Press, Boca Raton, FL, 2005, pp. 233–292.

[24] DuPont Medical Fabrics, *DuPont softesse.* Available at http://medicalfabrics.dupont.com/Medical_Fabrics/en_US/productServices/softess/index.html (accessed Aug 2010).

[25] R.F. Becker, E. Burgin, L.P.J. Burton and S.E. Amos, *Additive requirements for specific markets – medical applications,* Chap. 4.7, in *Polypropylene Handbook,* P. Nello, ed., Hanser, Munich, Germany, 2005.

[26] INDA Association of Nonwoven Fabrics Industry, *Medical drapes & gowns.* Available at http://www.inda.org/enduses/hlthbro/DrapesandGowns.html (accessed Aug 2010).

[27] C.O. Samuel and Uqbolue (eds.), *The use of polyolefins in industrial and medical applications,* Chap. 5, in *Polyolefin Fibres: Industrial and Medical Applications,* Woodhead, Cambridge, 2009, pp. 133–153.

[28] W.A. Rutala and D.J. Weber, Infect. Control Hosp. Epidemiol. 22(4) (2001, Apr) pp. 248–257. Available at http://www.unc.edu/depts/spice/dis/ICHE-2001-Apr-p248.pdf (accessed Aug 2010).

[29] E. Ghassemieh, M. Acar and H.K. Versteeg, Compos. Sci. Technol. 61(12) (2001, Sep) pp. 1681–1694.

[30] Cotton Incorporated, *Spunlaced or Hydroentangled Nonwovens,* Available at http://www.cottoninc.com/Cotton-Nonwoven-News/Spunlaced-Or-Hydroentangled-Nonwovens/ (accessed Oct 2010).

[31] L. Mario, R.M. Vasconcelos, M.J. Abreu and M.E. Cabeço Silva, *TEKSTiL ve KONFEKSiYON* 4 (2008) pp. 258–262.

[32] H.Y. Huang and X.M.G. Gao, *Spunlace (hydroentanglement),* updated by M.G. Kamath, A. Dahiya and R.R. Hegde, Apr 2004. Available at http://www.engr.utk.edu/mse/Textiles/Spunlace.htm (accessed Aug 2010).

[33] R.J. Wagner, *The Technical Needs – Nonwovens for Medical/Surgical and Consumer Uses,* D.F. Durso, ed., Tappi Press, Atlanta, GA, 1986, pp. 67–111.

[34] Y. Kim, *The use of polyolefins in industrial and medical applications,* Chap. 5, in *Polyolefin Fibres: Industrial and Medical Applications,* C.O.U. Samuel, ed., Woodhead, Cambridge, 2009.

[35] P. Nello (ed.), *Polypropylene Handbook,* Hanser, Munich, 2005.

[36] World Intellectual Property Organization (WIPO) IP Services, *UV stabilized outdoor cover with barrier properties (WO/2000/038914).* Available at http://www.wipo.int/pctdb/en/wo.jsp?IA=WO2000038914&DISPLAY=DESC (accessed Aug 2010).

[37] W. Albrecht, H. Fuchs and W. Kittelmann (eds.), *Nonwoven Fabrics*, Wiley-VCH, Weinheim, 2003.

[38] H. Rong and R. Kotra, *Wet-Laid Nonwovens*, updated by A. Dahiya, M.G. Kamath and R.R. Hegde (2004, Apr). Available at http://www.engr.utk.edu/mse/Textiles/Wet%20Laid%20Nonwovens.htm (accessed Oct 2010).

[39] L. Bergmann, Nonwovens Rep. Int. 4(10), 1995, p. 14.

[40] Indian Link Exchange, *Technical textiles and non wovens*. Available at http://sites.google.com/site/sekhonns/technicaltextilesandnonwovens (accessed Oct 2010).

[41] I.V. Walker, *Nonwovens – the choice for the medical industry into the next millennium*, Chap. 2, in *Medical Textiles: Proceedings of the International Conference 24 & 25 August 1999, Bolton, UK*, A. Subhash, ed., CRC Press, Boca Raton, FL, 2001.

[42] R.K. Virk, G.N. Ramaswamy, M. Bourham and B.L. Bures, Text. Res. J. 74(12) (2004, Dec) pp. 1073–1079.

[43] AAMI, *Selection of Surgical Gowns and Drapes in Health Care Facilities*, 2nd ed., Tech. Rep. 11, Association for the Advancement of Medical Instrumentation – Standards, Arlington, VA, 1994.

[44] M.S. Hubbard, K. Wadsworth, G.L. Telford and E.J. Quebbeman, AORN J. 55(1) (1992, Jan), pp. 194–201.

[45] C.G. Mayhall, *Hospital Epidemiology and Infection Control*, 3rd ed., Lippincott Williams & Wilkins, Philadelphia, PA, 2004.

[46] G.W. Scrivens, *Method of making apparel*, US Patent 4631756, 30 Dec, 1986.

[47] F.G. Lopez, *Medical gown with seamless sleeve protector*, US Patent 5444871, 29 Aug, 1995.

[48] R.M. Wheeler and J.A. Germy, *Protective hospital gown*, US Patent 4845779, 11 Jul, 1989.

[49] R.L. Holt, *Disposable surgical gown*, US Patent 5271100, 21 Dec, 1993.

[50] J.L. Taylor, C.A. Pinilla, J. Serrano and J.D. Hart, *Medical gown with an adhesive closure*, US Patent 6138278, 31 Oct, 2000.

[51] T. May-Plumlee and A. Pittman, J. Text. Apparel Technol. Manage. 2(2) (2002, Spring) pp. 1–9.

[52] C.A. Pissiotis, V. Komborozos, C. Papoutsi and G. Skrekas, Eur. J. Surg. 163(8) (1997, Aug) pp. 597–604.

[53] Center for Research on Textile Protection and Comfort (T-PACC), *Surgical Gown Wear Trials*, College of Textiles, North Carolina State University, NC, 1997.

[54] Center for Research on Textile Protection and Comfort (T-PACC), *Comfort Testing*, College of Textiles, North Carolina State University. Available at http://www.tx.ncsu.edu/tpacc/comfort/index.html (accessed Oct, 2010).

[55] N.L. Belkin, Infect. Cont. Hosp. Epidemiol. 15(11) (1994, Nov) pp. 713–716.

[56] B.J. Gruendemann, Infect. Control Today (2002, Mar). Available at http://www.kchealthcare.com/docs/takingcover.pdf (accessed Oct 2009).

[57] N.L. Belkin, Today's OR Nurse 16(4) (1994) pp. 5–7.

[58] W.C. Beck, N.L. Belkin and K.K. Meyer, Guthrie J. 63(2) (1994) pp. 73–76.

[59] W.C. Beck, N.L. Belkin and K.K. Meyer, Am. J. Surg. 169(3) (1995) pp. 286–287.

[60] H.C. Huang, C.H. Lee and S.L. Wu, J. Clin. Nurs. 15(4) (2006, Apr) pp. 436–443.

[61] M. Rhalimi, R. Helou and P. Jaecker, Drugs Aging 26(10) (2009) pp. 847–852.

[62] P. Kannus and J. Parkkari, Age Ageing 35(Suppl 2) (2006, Sep) pp. ii51–ii54.

[63] Q. Wang, J.W. Teo, A. Ghasem-Zadeh and E. Seeman, Osteoporos Int. 20(7) (2009, Jul) pp. 1151–1156.

[64] R.A. Marottoli, L.F. Berkman and L.M. Cooney, J. Am. Geriatr. Soc. 40 (1992) pp. 861–866.

[65] G.S. Keene, M.J. Parker and G.A. Pryor, BMJ 307(6914) (1993, Nov 13) pp. 1248–1250.

[66] F.D. Wolinsky, J.F. Fitzgerald and T.E. Stump, Am. J. Public Health 87(3) (1997, Mar) pp. 398–403.

[67] P. Kannus, J. Parkkari, S. Koskinen, S. Niemi, M. Palvanen, M. Järvinen and I. Vuori, JAMA 281(20) (1999, May 26) pp. 1895–1899.

[68] Patent Storm, *Hip protector*, US Patent 5584072. Available at http://www.patentstorm.us/patents/5584072/description.html (accessed Oct 2009).

[69] Wikipedia, the free encyclopedia. *Hip protector*. Available at http://en.wikipedia.org/wiki/Hip_protector (accessed Oct 2009).

[70] A.M. Sawka, P. Boulos, K. Beattie, L. Thabane, A. Papaioannou, A. Gafni, A. Cranney, N. Zytaruk, D.A. Hanley and J.D. Adachi, Osteoporos Int. 16(12) (2005, Dec) pp. 1461–1474.

[71] A.M. Sawka, P. Boulos, K. Beattie, A. Papaioannou, A. Gafni, A. Cranney, D.A. Hanley, J.D. Adachi, E.A. Papadimitropoulos and L. Thabane, J. Clin. Epidemiol. 61(8) (2008, Aug) p. 854.

[72] T. Koike, Y. Orito, H. Toyoda, M. Tada, R. Sugama, M. Hoshino, Y. Nakao, S. Kobayashi, K. Kondo, Y. Hirota and K. Takaoka, Osteoporos. Int. 20(9) (2009, Sep) pp. 1613–1620.

[73] F.S.F. Ng and P.C.L. Hui, *Medical garment: a modern perspective*. Proceedings of the 39th Textile Research Symposium at Indian Institute of Technology (IIT) Delhi, New Delhi, India, 2010, pp. 370–377.

[74] H. Meinander and M. Varheenmaa (2002), *VTT processes*. Available at http://www.vtt.fi/inf/pdf/tiedotteet/2002/T2143.pdf (accessed Oct 2009).

[75] M.J. Parker, W.J. Gillespie and L.D. Gillespie, Cochrane Database Syst. Rev. (3) (2005, Jul 20), CD001255.

[76] R. Tideiksaar, *Hip protectors*. Available at http://www.seekwellness.com/fallprevention/hip-protectors.htm (accessed Oct 2009).

[77] FreePatentsOnline, *Hip pad for protecting greater trochanter from impact*. Available at http://www.freepatentsonline.com/5717997.pdf (accessed Oct 2009).

[78] P. Kannus, J. Parkkari and J. Poutala, Bone 25(2) (1999) pp. 229–235.

[79] S. Heidi and L. Donna, *Hip protectors and community-living seniors: A review of the literature*. Available at http://aix1.uottawa.ca/~nedwards/chru/english/pdf/CHRU%20Monograph%20Series%20M04.04.pdf (accessed Oct 2009).

[80] S. Derler, A.B. Spierings and K.U. Schmitt, Med. Eng. Phys. 27(6) (2005, Jul) pp. 475–485.

[81] H. Bentzen, A. Bergland and L. Forsén, Inj. Prev. 14(5) (2008, Oct) pp. 306–310.

[82] N.M. van Schoor, A.J. van der Veen, L.A. Schaap, T.H. Smit and P. Lips, Bone 39(2) (2006, Aug) pp. 401–407.

[83] F. Nabhani and J. Bamford, J. Mater. Process Technol. 124(3) (2002, 20 Jun) pp. 311–318.

[84] J. Parkkari, P. Kannus, J. Heikkilä, J. Poutala, H. Sievänen and I. Vuori, J. Bone Miner. Res. 10(10) (1995 Oct) pp. 1437–1442.

[85] M. Schmid Daners, L. Wullschleger, S. Derler and K.U. Schmitt, Med. Eng. Phys. 30(9) (2008, Nov) pp. 1186–1192.

[86] I.D. Cameron, BMJ 324 (2002) pp. 375–376. Available at http://www.bmj.com/cgi/content/full/324/7334/375 (accessed Oct 2009).

[87] I.D. Cameron, J. Venman, S.E. Kurrle, K. Lockwood, C. Birks, R.G. Cumming, S. Quine and G. Bashford, Age Ageing 30(6) (2001, Nov) pp. 477–481.

[88] I.D. Cameron, R.G. Cumming, S.E. Kurrle, S. Quine, K. Lockwood, G. Salkeld and T. Finnegan, Injury Prev. 9(2) (2003, Jun) pp. 138–141.

[89] W. Zhong, A. Ahmad, M.M. Xing, P. Yamada and C. Hamel, Cutan. Ocul. Toxicol. 27(1) (2008) pp. 21–28.

[90] FreePatentsOnline, *Woven cotton-polyester blend fabrics having recoverable stretch characteristics*. Available at http://www.freepatentsonline.com/3290752.pdf (accessed Oct 2009).

[91] L.A. Honkanen, M.L. Dehner and M.S. Lachs, J. Am. Med. Dir. Assoc. 7(9) (2006, Nov) pp. 550–555.

[92] W.E. Wortberg, Zeitschrift fur Gerontologie 21(3) (1988, May–Jun) pp. 169–173.

[93] P. Jantti, H. Aho and L. Maki-Jokela, Suomen Lõõkõrilehti 51(32) (1996) pp. 3387–3389.

[94] J.B. Lauritzen, M.M. Pertersen and B. Lund, Lancet 341(8836) (1993, Jan 2) pp. 11–13.

[95] J. Parkkari, P. Kannus, J. Poutala and I. Vuori, J. Bone Miner. Res. 9(9) (1994, Sep) pp. 1391–1396.

[96] J. Woo, C. Sum, H.H. Yiu, K. Ip, L. Chung and L. Ho, Clin. Rehabil. 17(2) (2003, Mar) pp. 203–205.

[97] D. Torgerson and J. Porthouse, BMJ 326 (2003, 26 Apr) p. 930. Available at http://www.bmj.com/cgi/content/full/326/7395/930?maxtoshow=&HITS=10&hits=10&RESULTFORMAT=1&title=Effectiveness+of+hip+protectors+&andorexacttitle=and&andorexacttitleabs=and&andorexactfulltext=and&searchid=1&FIRSTINDEX=0&sortspec=relevance&volume=326&fdate=1/1/1981&resourcetype=HWCIT (accessed Oct 2009).

[98] M. Matarese and A. Picciacchia, Prof. Inferm. 59(2) (2006 Apr–Jun) pp. 109–118.

[99] M.T. Villar, P. Hill, H. Inskip, P. Thompson and C. Cooper, Age Ageing 27(2) (1998, Mar) pp. 89–90.

[100] C. Cryer, A. Knox, D. Martin, J. Barlow and Cantebury Hip Protector Project Team, Inj. Prev. 8(3) (2002, Sep) pp. 202–206.

[101] N.M. van Schoor, W.L. Devillé, L.M. Bouter and P. Lips, Osteoporos Int. 13(12) (2002, Dec) pp. 917–924.

[102] C.W. Fan, K.M. Tan, D. Coakley, J.B. Walsh and C. Cunningham, Ir. J. Med. Sci. 174(1) (2005, Jan–Mar) pp. 49–54.

[103] H. Jonathan, P. Elizabeth and K. Erin, J. Safety Res. 37(4) (2006) pp. 421–424.

[104] P. Kannus, J. Parkkari, S. Niemi, M. Pasanen, M. Palvanen, M. Järvinen and I. Vuori, N. Engl. J. Med. 21(343) (2000, Nov 23) pp. 1506–1513.

[105] T. Suzuki, H. Yoshida, T. Ishizaki, H. Yukawa, S. Watanabe, S. Kumagai, S. Shinkai, H. Shibata, T. Nakamura, S. Yasumura and H. Haga, Nippon Ronen Igakkai Zasshi 36(1) (1999, Jan) pp. 40–44.

[106] S. Yasumura, T. Suzuki, H. Yoshida, T. Ishizaki, H. Yukawa, S. Watanabe, S. Kumagai, H. Shibata, T. Nakamura, N. Niino, H. Haga, H. Imuta, H. Abe and A. Fukao, Nippon Ronen Igakkai Zasshi 36(4) (1999, Apr) pp. 268–273.

[107] D.K. Chan, G. Hillier, M. Coore, R. Cooke, R. Monk, J. Mills and W.T. Hung, Arch. Gerontol. Geriatr. 30(1) (2000, Jan–Feb) pp. 25–34.

[108] H. Bentzen, L. Forsén, C. Becker and A. Bergland, Osteoporos. Int. 19(1) (2008, Jan) pp. 101–111.

[109] J. Minns, F. Nabhani and J. Bamford, *How safe are hip protectors?* Available at http://www.rospa.com/homesafety/info/hip_protectors.pdf (accessed Oct 2009).

[110] L. Forsén, C. Arstad, S. Sandvig, A. Schuller, U. Røed and A.J. Søgaard, Scand. J. Public Health 31(4) (2003) pp. 261–266.

[111] C. Birks, K. Lockwood, I. Cameron, S. Kurrle, W. Burnside, S. Easter, J. Venman, R. Cumming, S. Quine, G. Salkeld and T. Finnegan, Australas. J. Ageing 18(1) (1999) pp. 23–26.

[112] H. Seo, S.J. Kim, F. Cordier and K. Hong, *Validating a cloth simulator for measuring tight-fit clothing pressure*, Proceedings of the 2007 ACM Symposium on Solid and Physical Modeling – ACM Symposium on Solid and Physical Modeling, Beijing, China, 4–6 June 2007, pp. 431–437. Available at http://www.rospa.com/homesafety/info/hip_protectors.pdf (accessed Oct 2009).

[113] N.M. van Schoor, G. Asma, J.H. Smit, L.M. Bouter and P. Lips, Osteoporos. Int. 14(4) (2003, Jun) pp. 353–359.

[114] M.L. Bouxsein, P. Szulc, F. Munoz, E. Thrall, Sornay-E. Rendu and P.D. Delmas, J. Bone Miner. Res. 22(6) (2007, Jun) pp. 825–831.

[115] R.J. Minns, A.M. Marsh, A. Chuck and J. Todd, Age Ageing 36(2) (2007, Mar) pp. 140–144.

[116] HipSaver, *EZ pull-up handles help for those with weakened grip-strength.* Available at http://www.hipsaver.com/models.html#ezpull (accessed Oct 2009).

[117] HipSaver, *Open crotch design for easy toileting.* Available at http://www.hipsaver.com/models.html#openbottom (accessed Oct 2009).

[118] HipSaver, *Incontinence management with wrap&snap.* Available at http://www.hipsaver.com/models.html#wrapnsnap (accessed Oct 2009).

[119] S. Guangyi, C. Cheung-Shing, L. Yilun, Z. Guanglie, J.L. Wen, H.W.L. Philip and L. Kwok-Sui, *Development of a human airbag system for fall protection using MEMS motion sensing technology.* Available at http://www2.acae.cuhk.edu.hk/~cmns/papers/IEEE-IROS-2006-gyshi.pdf (accessed Oct 2009).

[120] W.W. Reid, J.H. Evans, R.S. Naismith, A.E. Tully and S. Sherwin, Burns 13(Suppl) (1987) pp. S29–S32.

[121] S.W. Parry, Clin. Plast. Surg. 16(3) (1989 Jul) pp. 577–586.

[122] D.L. Larson, S. Abston, E.B. Evans, M. Dobrkovsky, B. Willis and H. Linares, *Development and correction of burn scar contracture*, in *Development and Correction of Burn Scar Contracture*, P. Matter, ed., 3rd International Congress for Research in Burns, Prague, Hans Hubber, Vienna, 1970.

[123] B.O. Mofikoya, W.L. Adeyemo and A.A. Abdus-Salam, Nig. Q. J. Hosp. Med. 17(4) (2007, Oct–Dec) pp. 134–739.

[124] B. Berman, M.H. Viera, S. Amini, R. Huo and I.S. Jones, J. Craniofac. Surg. 19(4) (2008, Jul) pp. 989–1006.

[125] D. Wolfram, A. Tzankov, P. Pülzl and H. Piza-Katzer, Dermatol. Surg. 35(2) (2009, Feb) pp. 171–181.

[126] R.S. Naismith, *Hypertrophic scar therapy pressure-induced remodelling and its determinants*, PhD thesis, Bioengineering Unit, Strathclyde University, Glasgow, UK, 1980.

[127] N. Yildiz, Burns 33(1) (2007, Feb) pp. 59–64.

[128] S. Ripper, B. Renneberg, C. Landmann, G. Weigel and G. Germann, Burns 35 (5) (2009, Aug) pp. 657–664.

[129] L. Macintyre and M. Baird, Burns 32(1) (2006) pp. 10–15.

[130] M.C. Spires, B.M. Kelly and P.H. Pangilinan, Jr., Phys. Med. Rehabil. Clin. N. Am. 18(4) (2007, Nov) pp. 925–948, viii.

[131] M.A. Haq and A. Haq, East Afr. Med. J. 67(11) (1990, Nov) pp. 785–793.

[132] M.J. Brennan and L.T. Miller, Cancer 83(12 Suppl. Am.) (1998, Dec 15) pp. 2821–2827.

[133] M. Arrault and S. Vignes, Bull. Cancer 94(7) (2007, Jul 1) pp. 669–674.

[134] R.B. Jordan, J. Daher and K. Wasil, Clin. Plast. Surg. 27(1) (2000, Jan) pp. 71–85.

[135] L. Macintyre and M. Baird, Burns 31(1) (2005, Feb) pp. 11–14.

[136] Mölnlycke Health Care, *Tubigrip elasticated tubular bandage.* Available at http://www.molnlycke.com/com/Wound-Care-Products/Product-selector—Wound-division/Tabs/Products/Tubigrip-Elasticated-Tubular-Bandage/?activeTab=2 (accessed Oct 2010).

[137] S. Cheng, A. Chan, S. Fong, M. Lam, A. Leung, P. Lee, J. Tsang, J. Wong and A. Wu, Burns 22(8) (1996, Dec) pp. 623–626.

[138] JOBST Compression Institute, *What is the JOBST compression institute?* Available at http://jobstcompressioninstitute.com/content-4.html (accessed Oct 2010).

[139] J.F. Annis and P. Webb, *Development of a Space Activity Suit. NASA Contractor Rep,* National Aeronautics and Space Administration, Washington, DC, Nov 1971.

[140] L.M. Macintyre and M.R. Baird, Burns 31(1) (2005) pp. 11–14.

[141] M. Manto, M. Topping, M. Soede, Sanchez-J. Lacuesta, W. Harwin, J. Pons, J. Williams, S. Skaarup and L. Normie, IEEE Eng. Med. Biol. Mag.22(3) (2003, May/June) pp. 120–132.

[142] Bio-Concepts, Inc., of Phoenix, Arizona, *Bio-concepts fabric materials.* Available at http://www.bio-con.com/materials.html (accessed Oct 2010).

[143] M.H. Malick and J.A. Carr, Am. J. Occup. Ther. 34(9) (1980, Sep) pp. 603–608.

[144] Z. Medical, *Custom-made burn garments.* Available at http://www.medicalz.com/burn-garments.htm (accessed Oct 2010).

[145] Z. Medical, *Custom made burn garments – standard fabric.* Available at http://www.medicalz.com/burn-garments-standard.htm (accessed Oct 2010).

[146] Z. Medical, *Custom made burn garments – coolmax fabric.* Available at http://www.medicalz.com/burn-garments-coolmax.htm (accessed Oct 2010).

[147] R. Casley-Smith Judith and J.R. Casley-Smith, *Suppliers of compression garments for the treatment of lymphedema.* Available at http://k-t.org/wp-content/uploads/2010/02/Compression-garments.pdf (accessed Oct 2010).

[148] S.F. Ng and C.L. Hui, Text. Res. J. 71(3) (2001, March) pp. 275–279.

[149] L. Macintyre, Burns 33(5) (2007, Aug) pp. 579–586.

[150] K.S. Leung, J.C.Y. Cheng, G.F.Y. Ma, J.A. Clark and P.C. Leung, Burns 10 (6) (1984, Aug) pp. 434–438.

[151] C.L. Hui and S.F. Ng, Text. Res. J. 71(8) (2001, Aug) pp. 683–687.

[152] S.C. Shrestha and J.R. Bell, *A wide strip tensile test of geotextiles.* Proceedings of The Second International Conference on Geotextiles, Las Vegas, 1982.

[153] S.F. Ng and C.L. Hui, Text. Res. J. 71(5) (2001, May) pp. 381–383.

[154] S.F. Ng, *Design of pressure garments for hypertrophic scar treatment,* PhD thesis, De Montfort University, Leicester, UK, Sep 1995.

[155] S.F.F. Ng and C.L.P. Hui, Int. J. Clothing Sci. Technol. 11(5) (1999) pp. 251–262.

[156] J.C.Y. Cheng, J.H. Evans, K.S. Leung, J.A. Clark, T.T.C. Choy and P.C. Leung, Burns 10(3) (1984, Feb) pp. 154–163.

[157] C.L. Hui and S.F. Ng, Text. Res. J. 73(3) (2003, Mar) pp. 268–272.

[158] UW Health, *Pressure garment information for burn patients.* Available at http://www.uwhealth.org/healthfacts/B_EXTRANET_HEALTH_INFORMATION-FlexMember-Show_Public_HFFY_1116944264137.html (accessed Oct 2010).

[159] F.S.F. Ng-Yip, Int. J. Clothing Sci. Technol. 6(4) (1994) pp. 17–27.

[160] B.G. Lamberty and J. Whitaker, Physiotherapy 67(1) (1981, Jan) pp. 2–4.

[161] F.S.F. Ng, *The properties and comfort of pressure garments for hypertrophic scar treatment,* MPhil thesis, Leicester Polytechnic, Leicester, UK, 1989.

[162] P.C. Leung and M. Ng, Burns 6(4) (1980, Jun) pp. 244–250.

[163] J.A. Carr-Collins, Clin. Plast. Surg. 19(3) (1992, Jul) pp. 733–743.

[164] M. Gibbons, R. Zuker, M. Brown, S. Candlish, L. Snider and P. Zimmer, J. Burn. Care Rehabil. 15(1) (199, Jan/Feb) pp. 69–73.

[165] C.L. Johnson, O'E.J. Shaughnessy and G. Ostergren, *Burn Management*, Raven Press, New York, NY, 1981, p. 2.

[166] F.S.F. Ng-Yip, Int. J. Clothing Sci. Technol. 5(1) (1993) pp. 17–24.

[167] R. Stewart, A.M. Bhagwanjee, Y. Mbakaza and T. Binase, Am. J. Occup. Ther. 54(6) (2000, Nov–Dec) pp. 598–606.

[168] J. Johnson, B. Greenspan, D. Gorga, W. Nagler and C. Goodwin, J. Burn Care Rehabil. 15(2) (1994, Mar–Apr) pp. 180–188.

[169] C.A. Brown, Burns 27(4) (2001, Jun) pp. 342–348.

[170] F. Williams, D. Knapp and M. Wallen, Burns 24(4) (1998) pp. 329–335.

[171] LegAids.com, *Jobst compression stockings.* Available at http://www.legaids.com/Jobst_Compression_Stockings.html (accessed Jan 2010).

[172] HubPages, *Compression stocking guide.* Available at http://hubpages.com/hub/Compression-Stockings (accessed Jan 2010).

[173] VNUS, *Venous reflux disease.* Available at http://www.vnus.com/venous-reflux/index.aspx (accessed Jan 2010).

[174] MedlinePlus, *Varicose veins.* Available at http://www.nlm.nih.gov/medlineplus/varicoseveins.html (accessed Jan 2010).

[175] B. Eklöf, R.B. Rutherford, J.J. Bergan, P.H. Carpentier, P. Gloviczki, R.L. Kistner, M.H. Meissner, G.L. Moneta, K. Myers, F.T. Padberg, M. Perrin, C.V. Ruckley, P.C. Smith, T.W. Wakefield and American Venous Forum International Ad Hoc Committee for Revision of the CEAP Classification, J. Vasc. Surg. 40(6) (2004, Dec) pp. 1248–1252.

[176] J.R. Stanton, E.D. Freis and R.W. Wilkins, J. Clin. Invest. 28(3) (1949, May) pp. 553–558.

[177] B.R. Meyerowitz and R. Nelson, Surgery 56 (1964, Sep) pp. 481–486.

[178] K. Ido, T. Suzuki, Y. Taniguchi, C. Kawamoto, N. Isoda, N. Nagamine, T. Ioka, K. Kimura, M. Kumagai and Y. Hirayama, Gastrointest. Endosc. 42(2) (1995, Aug) pp. 151–155.

[179] V. Ibegbuna, K.T. Delis, A.N. Nicolaides and O. Aina, J. Vasc. Surg. 37(2) (2003, Feb) pp. 420–425.

[180] O. Agu, D. Baker and A.M. Seifalian, Vascular 12(1) (2004, Jan) pp. 69–76.

[181] Fabric.com, *Fabric glossary.* Available at http://www.fabric.com/SitePages/Glossary.aspx (accessed Jan 2010).

[182] A.J. van Geest, J.C. Veraart, P. Nelemans and H.A. Neumann, Dermatol. Surg. 26(3) (2000, Mar) pp. 244–247.

[183] H.M. Häfner, M. Eichner and M. Jünger, Zentralbl. Chir. 126(7) (2001, Jul) pp. 551–556.

[184] R. Liu, Y.L. Kwok, Y. Li, T.T. Lao and X. Zhang, Fibers and Polym. 6(4) (2005) pp. 322–331.

[185] Z. Medical, *Custom made burn garments – Z grip fabric.* Available at http://www.medicalz.com/burn-garments-zgrip.htm (accessed Aug 2010).

[186] Laser Vein Center for Excellence, *Varicose veins & compression stockings information articles: The modern medical compression stockings.* Available at http://www.thelaserveincenter.com/articles#CVI (accessed Jan 2010).

[187] Ezine@rticles, *Different kinds of compression stockings.* Available at http://ezinearticles.com/?Different-Kinds-of-Compression-Stockings&id=5072007 (accessed Sep 2010).

[188] VienDirectory.org, *Compression stockings in Portland, Maine (ME).* Available at http://www.veindirectory.org/list/compression-stockings/Maine/Portland/2468/2 (accessed Jan 2010).

[189] What Health? *Compression stockings.* Available at http://www.whathealth.com/compressionstockings/index.html (accessed Jan 2010)

[190] LIVIT Orthopedie, *Medical compression stockings.* Available at http://www.livit.nl/medical-elastic-stockings-tek (accessed Jan 2010).

[191] BrightLife Direct, *Style or length.* Available at http://www.brightlifedirect.com/STYLE-OR-LENGTH/c356/index.html (accessed Jan 2010).

[192] BrightLife Direct, *A comprehensive guide to compression hosiery and compression hosiery manufacturers.* Available at http://www.brightlifedirect.com/which_brand_right.php (accessed Jan 2010).

[193] Wikipedia, the free encyclopedia, *Varicose veins.* Available at http://en.wikipedia.org/wiki/Varicose_veins (accessed Jan 2010).

[194] K.M. Zurat, Adv. Nurs. Pract. 11(6) (2003, Jun) pp. 1–6. Available at http://www. themedicalzone.com/assets/pdf_articles/varicose_veins_compression.pdf (accessed Jan 2010)

[195] R.H. Jones and P.J. Carek, Am. Fam. Physician 78(11) (2008, Dec 1) pp. 1289–1294.

[196] I. Lamberg Stanford, *Blackwell's Primary Care Essentials: Dermatology*, Blackwell Science, Malden, MA, 2002.

[197] W.S. Lam, Sci. Meet. 9(2) (2001, Jun) p. 85. Available at http://www.medicine. org.hk/hksdv/journal/200106-10.pdf (accessed Jan 2010).

[198] Eczema-Treatment-Guide.info (ETG), *Wet-wrap therapy for eczema, Eczema Treatment Guide*. Available at http://www.eczema-treatment-guide.info/wet-wrap-therapy-eczema.html (accessed Jan 2010).

[199] M.C. Stöppler, *Eczema*. MedicineNet.com. Available at http://www.medicinenet. com/eczema/article.htm (accessed Jan 2010).

[200] SkinCareWorld.co.uk, *Wet wrapping efficacy*, Mölnlycke Health Care Ltd. Available at http://www.skincareworld.co.uk/pharmacy/our_products/epaderm/WetWrappingEfficacy_ epaderm.htm#Ref2 (accessed Jan 2010).

[201] V. Iannelli, *Wet dressings for eczema*. About.com: Pediatrics. Available at http:// pediatrics.about.com/od/ezema/a/0408_wet_drsngs.htm (accessed Jan 2010).

[202] G.C. Sauer and J.C. Hall, *Manual of Skin Diseases*, Lippincott-Raven, Philadelphia, PA, 1996.

[203] L.A. Goldsmith, G.S. Lazarus and M.D. Tharp, *Adult and Pediatric Dermatology: A Color Guide to Diagnosis and Treatment*, F.A. Davis, Philadelphia, PA, 1997.

[204] T. Bieber and D.Y.M. Leung, *Atopic Dermatitis*, Marcel Dekker, New York, NY, 2002.

[205] The Royal Children's Hospital, Dermatology Department, *Wet dressings for eczema*. Available at http://www.rch.org.au/emplibrary/clinicalguide/Eczema_Wet_dressings.pdf (accessed Jan 2010).

[206] A.P. Oranje, A.C. Devillers, B. Kunz, S.L. Jones, L. DeRaeve, D. Van Gysel, F.B. de Waard-van der Spek, R. Grimalt, A. Torrelo, J. Stevens and J. Harper, J. Eur. Acad. Dermatol. Venereol. 20(10) (2006, Nov) pp. 1277–1286.

[207] U. Wollina, M.B. Abdel-Naser and S. Verma, Curr. Probl. Dermatol. 33 (2006) pp. 1–16.

[208] A. Kramer, P. Guggenbichler, P. Heldt, M. Jünger, A. Ladwig, H. Thierbach, U. Weber and G. Daeschlein, Curr. Probl. Dermatol. 33 (2006) pp. 78–109.

[209] M. Heide, U. Möhring, R. Hänsel, M. Stoll, U. Wollina and B. Heinig, Curr. Probl. Dermatol. 33 (2006) pp. 179–199.

[210] A. Gauger, S. Fischer, M. Mempel, T. Schaefer, R. Foelster-Holst, D. Abeck and J. Ring, J. Eur. Acad. Dermatol. Venereol. 20(5) (2006, May) pp. 534–541.

[211] A.B. Lansdown, Curr. Probl. Dermatol. 33 (2006) pp. 17–34.

[212] S. Haug, A. Roll, P. SchmidGrendelmeier, P. Johansen, B. Wüthrich, T.M. Kündig and G. Senti, Curr. Probl. Dermatol. 33 (2006) pp. 144–151.

[213] A. Gauger, Curr. Probl. Dermatol. 33 (2006) pp. 152–164.

[214] DermaSilk, *Features & benefits*. Available at http://www.dermasilk.co.uk/benefits.htm (accessed Jul 2010).

[215] S. Sarovart, B. Sudatis, P. Meesilpa, B.P. Grady and R. Magaraphan, Rev. Adv. Mater. Sci. 5 (2003) pp. 193–198.

[216] S. Terada, K. Yanagihara, K. Kaito, M. Miki, M. Sasaki, K. Tsujimoto and H. Yamada, Anim. Cell Technol. Meet. Genomics 2 (2005) pp. 585–587.

[217] R. Mason, J. Fam. Health Care 18(2) (2008) pp. 63–65.

[218] G. Ricci, A. Patrizi, F. Bellini and M. Medri, Curr. Probl. Dermatol. 33 (2006) pp. 127–143.

[219] H.M. Goodyear, K. Spowart and J.I. Harper, Br. J. Dermatol. 125 (1991) p. 604.

[220] W.E. Love and S.T. Nedorost, Dermatitis 20(1) (2009, Jan–Feb) pp. 29–33.

[221] SkinCareWorld.co.uk, *Frequently asked questions about Epaderm, Tubifast bandages and tubifast garments*. Available at http://www.skincareworld.co.uk/scw/faq.nsf/home? openform&s=ph&c=Product (accessed Jan 2010).

[222] A.C. Devillers and A.P. Oranje, Br. J. Dermatol. 154(4) (2006, Apr) pp. 579–585.

[223] B. Page, Br. J. Nurs. 14(5) (2005, Mar 10–23) pp. 289–290, 292.

[224] K.L. Hon, K.Y. Wong, L.K. Cheung, G. Ha, M.C. Lam, T.F. Leung, C.M. Chow, Y.M. Tang, N.M. Luk and A.K. Leung, J. Dermatol. Treat. 18(5) (2007) pp. 301–305.

[225] The Royal Children's Hospital Melbourne, *Wet dressings for eczema*. Knowing Your Child's Eczema. Available at http://wch.org.au/derm/eczema.cfm?doc_id=4596#Wet_Dressings_ (accessed Jan 2010).

[226] A.C.A. Devillers and A.P. Oranje, Br. J. Dermatol. 154(4) (2006, Apr) pp. 579–585.

[227] R. McGowan, P. Tucker, D. Joseph, A.M. Wallace, I. Hughes, N.P. Burrows and S.F. Ahmed, J. Dermatol. Treat. 14(3) (2003, Sep) pp. 149–152.

[228] K.L. Hon, T.F. Leung, Y. Wong, W.K. Lam, D.Q. Guan, K.C. Ma, Y.T. Sung, T.F. Fok and P.C. Leung, Am. J. Chin. Med. 32(6) (2004) pp. 941–950.

[229] M.J. Zohuriaan-Mehr and K. Kabiri, Iran Polym. J. 17(6) (2008) pp. 451–477.

[230] F.L. Buchholz and A.T. Graham, *Modern Superabsorbent Polymer Technology*, Wiley-VCH, New York, NY, 1998.

[231] R.P. Teli and P.D. Pardeshi, Indian Text. J. 111(9) (2001, Sep) pp. 15–26 (Bombay, India: Business Press Private Ltd.).

[232] Vincent P. Laake. *Substrates comprising flocked fibres of superabsorbent polymer*. US Patent No. 2004/0137191A1. Filing date: 23 Dec 2003.

[233] P. Akers and R. Heath, *Superabsorbent fibers: key to a new generation of medical nonwovens*, Nonwovens Rep. International, 1996, p. 305.

[234] S. Davies, *Text. Horiz.* 8(2) (1998) p. 18 (The International Magazine of the Textile Institute, Manchester, UK).

[235] S.A. Ceca, C. Gancet, S. Nicolas and K. Taupin, World Text. Abstr. 32(1) (2000) EP0938347.

[236] R.I. Shekar, A.K. Yadav, K. Kumar and V.S. Tripathi, Man-Made Text. India 46(12) (2003) pp. 9–16.

[237] E.D. Thompson, J.L. Seymour, M.J. Aardema, R.A. LeBoeuf, B.L. Evans and D.B. Cody, Environ. Mol. Mutagen. 18(3) (1991) pp. 184–199.

[238] R.C. Lindenschmidt, L.C. Stone, J.L. Seymour, R.L. Anderson, P.A. Forshey and M.J. Winrow, Fundam. Appl. Toxicol. 17(1) (1991, Jul) pp. 128–135.

[239] A.T. Lane, P.A. Rehder and K. Helm, Am. J. Dis. Child. 144(3) (1990, Mar) pp. 315–318.

[240] M.D. Sobsey, C. Wallis and J.L. Melnick, Appl. Microbiol. 30(4) (1975, Oct) pp. 565–574.

[241] M. Huber, C. Gerba, M. Abbaszadegan, J. Robinson and S. Bradford, Environ. Sci. Technol. 28 (9) (1994) pp. 1767–1772.

[242] B.E. Rittmann, J.A. Sutfin and B. Henry, Biodegradation 2(3) (1991–1992) pp. 181–191.

[243] S.A. Weerawarna, *Biodegradable superabsorbent particles containing cellulose fiber*, Seattle, WA, US Patent – Pub. No. 2009/0326180 A1. Available at http://www.freepatentsonline. com/20090326180.pdf (accessed Aug 2010).

[244] Q. Yimin, J. Text. Inst. 92(2) (2001) pp. 127–138.

[245] Duncan Mortimer, *Moist wound dressings and pressure relieving surfaces*, The Centre for Health Program Evaluation (CHPE). Available at http://cms-public.buseco.monash.edu.au/centres/che/pubs/wp104.pdf (accessed Aug 2010).

[246] V. Jones and T. Milton, Nursing times.net. 96 (45) (2000, 9 Nov) p. 2.

[247] Y. Qin, Int. Wound J. 2(2) (2005, Jun) pp. 172–176.

[248] G. Lee, S.C. Anand, S. Rajendran and I. Walker, J. Wound Care 15(8) (2006, Sep) pp. 344–346.

[249] B. Liesenfeld, D. Moore, A. Mikhaylova, J. Vella, R. Carr, G. Schultz and G. Olderman (2009), *Antimicrobial wound dressings: Mechanisms and Function*, QuickMed Technol. (QMT) 2005 SAWC. Available at http://www.quickmedtech.com/downloads/pdfs/2009%2004%20SAWC%20antimicrobial%20dressings_mech%20and%20func.pdf (accessed Aug 2010).

[250] S. Rajendran, *Antimicrobial textile dressings in managing wound infection – Qin Y, Jiaxing College, China*, Ch. 7, in *Advanced Textiles for Wound Care*, Woodhead, Oxford, 2009.

[251] P. Lu and B. Ding, Recent. Pat. Nanotechnol. 2(3) (2008) pp. 169–182.

[252] S. Rajendran, *Interactive dressings and their role in moist wound management – Weller C, Monash University, Australia*, Ch. 4, in *Advanced Textiles for Wound Care*. Woodhead, Oxford, 2009.

[253] L. Van Langenhove, *Smart wound care materials – Qin Y, Jiaxing College, China*, Ch. 2, in *Smart Textiles for Medicine and Healthcare: Materials, Systems and Applications*, Woodhead, Cambridge, 2007.

[254] M. Fader, A.M. Cottenden and K. Getliffe, Cochrane Database Syst. Rev. (4) (2008, Oct 8) CD007408.

[255] M. Fader, A.M. Cottenden and K. Getliffe, Cochrane Database Syst. Rev. (2) (2007, Apr 18) CD001406.

[256] Answer.com, *How is a disposable diaper made?* Available at http://www.answers.com/topic/disposable-diaper (accessed Aug 2010).

[257] Wikipedia, the free encyclopedia, *Diaper.* Available at http://en.wikipedia.org/wiki/Diaper (accessed Aug 2010).

[258] Gladwell.com, Ann. Technol. (2001, Nov 26). Available at http://www.gladwell.com/2001/2001_11_26_a_diaper.htm (accessed Aug 2010).

[259] C.F. White, Proc. Inst. Mech. Eng. H. 217(4) (2003) pp. 243–251.

[260] The Diaper Industry Source, *What are the components of a typical disposable diaper?* Available at http://www.disposablediaper.net/faq.asp?1 (accessed Aug 2010).

[261] M.D. Teli and N. Verma, Man-Made Text. India 32(7) (1989) p. 268.

[262] R. Nagaswarna, *Overview of disposable diaper parts and their purpose – absorbent core – wood pulp fluff.* Available at http://www.fibre2fashion.com/industry-article/12/1124/overview-of-disposable-diaper-parts-and-their-purpose3.asp (accessed Aug 2010).

[263] Anon, Synth. Fibres 29(1) (2000) p. 19.

[264] F.M. Lee, *Diaper visual indicator*, US Patent 5947943. Available at http://www.freepatentsonline.com/5947943.pdf (accessed Aug 2010).

[265] M.E. Brink, *Diaper with fastener*, US Patent 3618608. Available at http://www.freepatentsonline.com/3618608.pdf (accessed Aug 2010).

[266] C.E. Warnken, *Belted diapers*, US Patent 3653381. Available at http://www.freepatentsonline.com/3653381.pdf (accessed Aug 2010).

[267] R. Yamaki and K. Hisada, *Pull-on disposable diaper*, US Patent 5858012. Available at http://www.freepatentsonline.com/5858012.pdf (accessed Aug 2010).

[268] M. Fader, A. Cottenden, K. Getliffe, H. Gage, S. Clarke-O'Neill, K. Jamieson, N. Green, P. Williams, R. Brooks and J. Malone-Lee, Health Technol. Assess. 12(29) (2008 Jul) pp. iii–iv, ix–185.

[269] L. Van Langenhove and C. Hertleer, Int. J. Cloth. Sci. Technol. 16(1/2) (2004, Feb) pp. 63–72.

[270] F. Axisa, P.M. Schmitt, C. Gehin, G. Delhomme, E. McAdams and A. Dittmar, IEEE Trans. Inf. Technol. Biomed. 9(3) (2005, Sep) pp. 325–336.

[271] D. De Rossi, F. Lorussi, A. Mazzoldi, P. Orsini and E.P. Scilingo, *Monitoring body kinematics and gesture through sensing fabrics.* Proceedings of the 1st annual International IEEE–EMBS Special Topic Conference on Microtechnology, 12–14 Oct., 2000, p. 587.

[272] D. De Rossi, A. Mazzoldi, A. Dittmar and L. Schwenzfeier, *DRESSWARE: Smart fabrics and interactive clothing.* Proceedings of the 4th Workshop of Multifunctional Smart Polymer Systems, Sep. 1999, pp. 20–23.

[273] C. Lauterbach and S. Jung, *Integrated microelectronics for smart textiles*, in *Ambient Intelligence*, Springer, Berlin, Heidelberg, 2005, pp. 31–47.

[274] J. Turner and NASA, Ind. Prod. Manuf. Technol. (2006, Spinoff). Available at http://www.sti.nasa.gov/tto/Spinoff2006/ip_7.html (accessed Aug 2010).

[275] S. Carosio and A. Monero, Stud. Health Technol. Inform. 108 (2004) pp. 335–343.

[276] R. Paradiso and D. De Rossi, *Advances in textile sensing and actuation for e-textile applications.* Conference Proceedings of IEEE in Medicine and Biology Society, 2008, p. 3629.

[277] R. Paradiso, G. Loriga, N. Taccini, A. Gemignani and C. Belloc, J. Telecommun. Inform. Tech. 9(3) (4/2005) pp. 105–113.

[278] M. Pacelli, G. Loriga, N. Taccini and R. Paradiso, *Sensing fabrics for monitoring physiological and biomechanical variables: e-textile solutions.* Proceedings of the 3rd IEEE-EMBS, 6 Sep. 2006, pp. 1–4.

[279] X Tao, Text. Asia (Jan. 2002) pp. 38–41.

[280] A.M. da Rocha, Stud. Health Technol. Inform. 108 (2004) pp. 330–334.

[281] D. Raskovic, T. Martin and E. Jovanov, Comput. J. 47(4) (2004) pp. 495–504.

[282] S. Park, C. Gopalsamy, R. Rajamanickam and S. Jayaraman, Stud. Health Technol. Inform. 62 (1999) pp. 252–258.

[283] C. Gopalsamy, S. Park, R. Rajamanickam and S. Jayaraman, Virtual Real. 4(3) (1999) pp. 152–168.

[284] Sensatex, *Sensatex seamless technology.* Available at http://www.sensatex.com/press/Wolf10-15-04.pdf (accessed Aug 2010).

[285] Sensatex, *Smart textile systems.* Available at http://www.sensatex.com/index.html (accessed Aug 2010).

[286] Sensatex, *SmartShirt system.* Available at http://www.sensatex.com/smartshirt.html (accessed Aug 2010).

[287] JERA (2006), *New "SmartShirt" uses nanotechnology to monitor heart rate, other vital signs in real time*, M2 Communications Ltd. Available at http://www.sensatex. com/press/mediaplacement.pdf (accessed Aug 2010).

[288] P. Lukowicz, U. Anliker, J. Ward, G. Tröster, E. Hirt and C. Neufelt, *AMON: A wearable medical computer for high-risk patient.* Proceedings of the 6th International Symposium on Wearable Computers, (ISWC 2002), The IEEE computer society, 7–10 Oct 2002, Seattle, Washington, USA.

[289] U. Anliker, J.A. Ward, P. Lukowicz, G. Tröster, F. Dolveck, M. Baer, F. Keita, E.B. Schenker, F. Catarsi, L. Coluccini, A. Belardinelli, D. Shklarski, M. Alon, E. Hirt, R. Schmid and M. Vuskovic, IEEE Trans. Inf. Technol. Biomed. 8(4) (2004, Dec) pp. 415–427.

[290] M. Di Rienzo, F. Rizzo, P. Meriggi, B. Bordoni, G. Brambilla, M. Ferratini and P. Castiglioni, *Applications of a textile-based wearable system for vital signs monitoring.* Proceedings of the 28th IEEE Engineering in Medicine and Biology Society Annual International Conference, New York City, NY, 30 Aug–3 Sep, 2006, pp. 2223–2226.

[291] M. Di Rienzo, F. Rizzo, G. Parati, G. Brambilla, M. Ferratini and P. Castiglioni, *MagIC system: A new textile-based wearable device for biological signal monitoring. Applicability in daily life and clinical setting.* Proceedings of the 2005 IEEE Engineering in Medicine and Biology 27th Annual Conference, Shanghai, China, 1–4 September, 2005, pp. 7167–7169.

[292] M. Di Rienzo, F. Rizzo, G. Parati, M. Ferratini, G. Brambilla and P. Castiglioni, Comput. Cardiol. 32 (2005) pp. 699–701.

[293] P. Augustyniak, Comput. Recogn. Syst. 30 (2005) pp. 469–476 (Springer, Berlin/Heidelberg).

[294] R. Tollen and Tech TV. *LifeShirt and smart shirt – wired garments monitor vital signs,* 19 Sep, 2001. Available at http://dev.binaryinteractive.com:8102/docs/press/techtv_20020129.pdf (accessed Jul 2010).

[295] N. Halín, M. Junnila, P. Loula and P. Aarnio, J. Telemed. Telecare. 11(Suppl. 2) (2005) pp. S41–S43.

[296] Talk about sleep, *VivoMetrics' LifeShirt system for monitoring patients at work, play and sleep,* Ventura, CA – 12 December, 2001. Available at http://www.talkaboutsleep.com/sleep-disorders/archives/Snoring_apnea_lifeshirt.htm (accessed Jul 2010).

[297] MEDES – Télémédecine, *VTAMN PROJECT (RNTS 2000): "Medical teleassistance suit."* Available at http://www.medes.fr/home_fr/telemedecine/assistance_aux_personnes/vtamn.html (accessed Aug 2010).

[298] N. Noury, A. Dittmar, C. Corroy, R. Baghai, J.L. Weber, D. Blanc, F. Klefstat, A. Blinovska, S. Vaysse and B. Comet, Conf. Proc. IEEE Eng. Med. Biol. Soc. 5 (2004) pp. 3266–3269.

[299] N. Noury, A. Dittmar, C. Corroy, R. Baghai, J.L. Weber, D. Blanc, F. Klefstat, A. Blinovska, S. Vaysse and B. Comet, Conf. Proc. IEEE (2004) pp. 155–160.

[300] J.E. McKenzie, Conf. Proc. IEEE Eng. Med. Biol. Soc. (2009) pp. 6882–6884.

[301] P. van de Ven, A. Bourke, J. Nelson and G. ÓLaighin, *A wearable wireless platform for fall and mobility monitoring.* Proceedings of the 1st International Conference on PErvasive Technologies Related to Assistive Environments, 2008, vol. 282, article 48.

[302] M.N. Boulos, A. Rocha, A. Martins, M.E. Vicente, A. Bolz, R. Feld, I. Tchoudovski, M. Braecklein, J. Nelson, G.O. Laighin, C. Sdogati, F. Cesaroni, M. Antomarini, A. Jobes and M. Kinirons, Int. J. Health Geogr. 6 (2007, Mar 12) pp. 1–6.

[303] ICT for Health – European Commission – Information Society and D.G. Media, *CAALYX: Increasing older people's autonomy and self-confidence.* Health Monthly Focus (2009, Oct) p. 1–2. Available at http://ec.europa.eu/information_society/activities/health/docs/monthly_focus/200910caalyx.pdf (accessed Aug 2010).

[304] H. Harms, O. Amft, G. Tröster and D. Roggen, *SMASH: A distributed sensing and processing garment for the classification of upper body postures.* Proceedings of the ICST 3rd International Conference on Body Area Networks, 2008, article 22.

[305] H. Harms, O. Amft and G. Tröster, *Influence of a loose-fitting sensing garment on posture recognition in rehabilitation.* Proceedings of IEEE Biomedical Circuits and Systems Conference, 2008, pp. 353–356.

[306] J. Sidén, A. Koptioug and M. Gulliksson, Microwave Symp. Digest, 2004 IEEE MTT-S Int. 2(6–11) (2004, Jun) pp. 659–662.

[307] Association for Automatic Identification and Mobility (AIM), *The "Smart" diaper moisture detection system.* Available at http://www.aimglobal.org/technologies/RFID/what_is_rfid.asp (accessed Aug 2010).

[308] L. Yambem, M.K. Yapici and J. Zou, IEEE Sensors J. 8(3) (2008, Mar) pp. 238–239.

[309] C.H. Yang, J.H. Chien, B.Y. Wang, P.H. Chien and D.S. Lee, Biomed. Microdevices 10(1) (2007) pp. 47–54.

[310] J. Siden, A. Koptioug and M. Gulliksson, Microwave Symp. Digest, 2004 IEEE MTT-S Int. 2 (2004, Jun) pp. 659–662.

[311] C.H. Yang, J.H. Chien and B.Y. Wang, Biomed. Microdevices 10 (2008) pp. 47–54.

[312] Q. Darren (2009), *Robotics*. Available at http://www.gizmag.com/robot-suit-hal/11471/ (accessed May 2010).

[313] D. Cory (2007), *Permalink*. Available at http://www.boingboing.net/2007/02/16/inflatable-exoskelet.html (accessed May 2010).

[314] S.Y. Cheng, C.W. Yuen, C.W. Kan, K.L.K. Cheuk, C.H. Chui and K.H. Lam, *Cosmetic textiles with biological benefits: Gelatin microcapsules containing Vitamin C*. Int. J. Mol. Med. Vol. 24, no. 4, October 2009, pp. 411–419.

[315] J. Koo and R. Desai, Dermatol. Ther. 16(2) (2003) pp. 98–105.

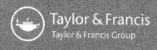
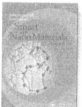
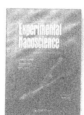
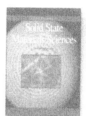
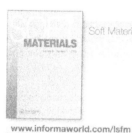
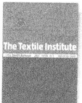
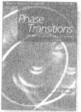
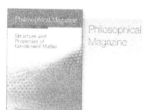
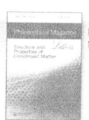

Instructions for Authors

General Style: Contributions suitable for *Textile Progress* should provide a critical and comprehensive examination of the subject matter. For most topics, a manuscript should cover the last five to ten years, using earlier relevant volumes of *Textile Progress* as a starting point. For more specialized or newer material that has not been covered previously in *Textile Progress*, it may be useful to take an earlier starting point.

Contributions should be written in such a way that they allow the non-specialist to understand the principles and applications of the topic. Articles should be broadly based and practically oriented. The appropriate style is that of a monograph, rather than that of a research paper or news article.

Contributions should aim to conform to a printed extent of 48 pp (including tables and illustrations), i.e. approximately 100 manuscript pages. If you feel that the subject requires a longer contribution, please discuss this with the Editor.
Manuscripts should include an appropriate list of references that will allow use as a resource for further study.

Submission of Manuscripts: Prospective authors are invited to submit an outline of their proposed contribution for consideration to:

Professor Xiaoming Tao, Editor-in-Chief,
Textile Progress, Institute of Textiles and Clothing,
Hong Kong Polytechnic University, Hung Hom, Kowloon,
Hong Kong. Email: tctaoxm@polyu.edu.hk.

Except under exceptional circumstances, text, tables and figures should be submitted electronically, along with hardcopy printouts for verification. Tables, figures and text should exist as separate files. *Do not embed either tables or figures in the text.* File names should be self-evident. Files may be prepared using Microsoft Word or LaTex. Please submit a pdf version of your article as well as the LaTex files.

The *Textile Progress* considers all manuscripts on the strict condition that they have been submitted only to the *Textile Progress* on this occasion and that they have not been published already, nor are they under consideration for publication or in press elsewhere. Authors who fail to adhere to this condition will be charged with all costs which *Textile Progress* incurs and their papers will not be published.

Language of Publication: Manuscripts must be written in English. The manuscript will be published in that version of standard English presented by the Author.

Specific Style Guidelines: Informative sub-headings should be used to divide the text. Manuscripts should start with a Table of Contents, in which the major topics are numbered 1., 2., etc., and the major subheadings are numbered 1.1, 1.2 etc. Minor subheadings are numbered 1.1.1,.1.1.2, etc. and 1.1.1.1, 1.1.1.2, etc., if needed. This system should be duplicated in the text of the article. Refer to recent issues of *Textile Progress* for examples.

Tables, figures, and equations are numbered sequentially, starting from 1, without regard to the topic and subhead numbering system. All numbering uses Arabic numerals.

References: References are indicated by bracketed numerals, e.g. [23], [23-26] or [23, 24, 27], starting from 1. In the Reference section, which is the last section of the manuscript, references are listed in consecutive numerical order.

Full reference style details are available on the Textile Progress homepage at www.tandf.co.uk/journals/TTPR.

Figures: Graphs and diagrams should be computer generated when possible and should be supplied in TIF or JPEG format at a resolution of 1200 dpi at their final size. Hard copy graphs and diagrams should be drawn in black ink on good quality paper or supplied as sharp glossy prints. If black-and-white halftones are to be included, the original photographs must be supplied with the manuscript. If originals are not available, electronic files should be supplied at a resolution of 300 dpi at their final size.
If figures are taken from previous publications it is the responsibility of the author to obtain the necessary written permission from the publisher concerned.

A list of captions for figures, including their attribution, if any, must be included. Label each figure on the back with the figure number and the name of the main authors. Illustrations will be reproduced in black and white.

Offprints: Authors will receive 50 free reprints, free online access to their article through our website (www.informaworld.com) and 5 complimentary copies of the issue containing their article. Complimentary reprints are available through Rightslink® and additional reprints can be ordered through Rightslink® when proofs are received. If you have any queries, please contact our reprints department at reprints@tandf.co.uk

Page charges: There are no page charges to individuals or institutions.

Printed and bound by CPI Group (UK) Ltd, Croydon, CR0 4YY

23/10/2024

01777685-0010